Water Fitness After 40

Ruth Sova

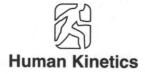

Human Kinetics

Library of Congress Cataloging-in-Publication Data

Sova, Ruth.
  Water fitness after 40 / Ruth Sova.
    p. cm.
  Includes bibliographical references and index.
  ISBN: 0-87322-604-6 (paper)
  1. Aquatic exercises. I. Title.
  GV838.53.E94S69 1995
  613.7'16--dc20   95-8270
                                                            CIP

ISBN: 0-87322-604-6

Developmental Editors: Glennda Kouts, Holly Gilly; **Assistant Editor:** Kirby Mittelmeier; **Copyeditor:** Margaret Harpool; **Proofreader:** Donna Brophy; **Indexer:** Margie Towery; **Typesetting and Layout:** Ruby Zimmerman; **Text Designer:** Stuart Cartwright; **Cover Designer:** Jack Davis; **Photo Editor:** Boyd LaFoon; **Photographer (cover):** Dale Wittner; **Photographer (interior):** Terry Wild Studio; **Illustrator:** Susan Carson; **Printer:** United Graphics

Human Kinetics books are available at special discounts for bulk purchase. Special editions or book excerpts can also be created to specification. For details, contact the Special Sales Manager at Human Kinetics.

Printed in the United States of America   10 9 8 7 6 5 4 3 2 1

Human Kinetics
P.O. Box 5076, Champaign, IL 61825-5076
1-800-747-4457
Canada: Human Kinetics, Box 24040, Windsor, ON N8Y 4Y9
1-800-465-7301 (in Canada only)
Europe: Human Kinetics, P.O. Box IW14, Leeds LS16 6TR, United Kingdom
(44) 1132 781708
Australia: Human Kinetics, 2 Ingrid Street, Clapham 5062, South Australia
(08) 371 3755
New Zealand: Human Kinetics, P.O. Box 105-231, Auckland 1
(09) 523 3462

CONTENTS

PREFACE

This book can help improve your fitness for the rest of your life. That's not just another sales pitch—it's true! As our life spans become longer, some form of exercise seems necessary so we can enjoy health and productivity throughout our lives. If you're over 40 and biology is starting to creep up on you, this book will help you slow that process. You don't need any special knowledge, and you don't have to be coordinated or have any special physical skills. All you need is you, this book, and a pool.

Most of us think that our bodies deteriorate naturally with age and that the deterioration is unavoidable. Now we're finding that discriminating between the effects of aging and the effects of inactivity is virtually impossible. No one should stop exercising or be afraid to start because he or she is too old.

I wrote this book because, like yours, my body is aging. I've looked for ways to stay in good health, but many of them cause more problems than they cure. Water exercise finally helped me, and I want it to help you, too. The benefits of exercise and the benefits of water work together to help offset the natural aging process and make our lives more enjoyable and productive.

In this book I've given you a few different approaches. Those of you who are interested in the background of water fitness and exercise in general will find that information in the first few chapters. Those of you who just want to jump in the pool and get going can use the workout chapters. I've provided guidelines for choosing a class and directions for creating your own program.

Do you need motivation? Read chapter 1. It describes the many benefits of water exercise, and it will get you moving. If you start to get in a rut, reread it.

Are you just beginning to exercise or are you already in great shape? Chapter 4 has programs for both situations and every one in between. Choose the workout that suits your fitness level and jump in. When you're ready for a change, try some of the other programs in this chapter.

Are you already happy with your aerobic workouts but need some extra toning to tighten up loose skin? Chapter 6 will tell you how to become sleek and firm.

Are you just finishing physical therapy? You can continue to improve with the postrehabilitation workout in chapter 7.

Do you have special medical concerns or physical limitations? You can still work out in the pool. Chapter 9 will tell you how to work with your special needs. It covers exercise modifications for arthritis, fibromyalgia, osteoporosis, shoulder problems, knee and hip problems, lower back pain, obesity, diabetes, coronary artery disease, hypertension, stroke, asthma and other breathing disorders, and gastrointestinal problems.

Chet Bradley, Executive Director of the Wisconsin Governor's Council on Physical Fitness, often says at our meetings, "If we don't change directions, we're liable to end up where we're going." Many of us want to be healthy, but too often we're going in the wrong direction to achieve that goal. You'll be setting some goals for yourself with the help of this book so you'll know the right direction. The exercise logs in chapter 10 should help you stay on track. Be sure to use them. They make a difference.

In case you're so motivated that you want to go further, the appendix lists organizations, other books, videos, and music that might interest you. I've also included sources for water exercise equipment and easy-to-wear aquatic apparel.

If you want to improve your life, have more energy to enjoy your grandchildren or another round of golf, run a marathon or take up water skiing, or have better self-esteem and a better outlook, this book can help you. The best part is that water exercise feels so good and is so much fun at the same time it's helping you meet your goals.

Read on, and start your adventure!

This book is for The Rev. Dr. and Mrs. R.J. Jalkanen, who taught me humility, perseverance, humor and the importance of education. Thank you for the unconditional love.

ACKNOWLEDGMENTS

None of my books have been written during tranquil times in my life. This leads me to believe there are no tranquil times. Therefore, I must thank those who brought me tranquillity during the writing of this book. Vicki Chossek who ran the Aquatic Exercise Association and then our new company, the Aquatic Therapy and Rehab Institute, while I wrote. Ellen Dybdahl and my daughter, Nicole, who took the dictaphone tape out of my hand and made the words come out on paper. Dave Garacci, my son-in-law and computer whiz who found everything I lost in the old computer and put it in the new computer. Kurt, my son, who stuck to his studies so I could stick to mine. Mary Schmit, Peggy Bannon and Maria Kiesow who not only picked up some of my personal obligations but who also read proofs and gave me ideas. Anne Miller and Paul and John Jalkanen who listened and listened and listened. . . . And special thanks to my husband, Bud, who willingly shopped or took me out to dinner when there was no food in the house. Most of all, I must thank Ted Miller and Holly Gilly at Human Kinetics who stuck with me through all my personal upheavals and made order out of chaos. Family and friends *are* God's way of loving us from afar.

Ruth Sova

FOREWORD

Ruth Sova personifies water fitness! Her love of helping people and her enjoyment of the water combine to form the underlying current of this book. With *Water Fitness After 40* you can begin splashing your way toward a healthier, happier lifestyle. Everything you need (except the pool) can be found in these pages: sensible advice, personal success stories, motivational suggestions, and exercises for every aspect of water fitness.

One of the greatest benefits of water exercise is that nearly everyone can participate in it. Regardless of age, ability level, or physical condition, people find that water provides a comfortable yet challenging environment in which to exercise. No longer does it matter if we are all on the same foot, if our figures are less than perfect, or if we need to move a little more slowly. The water encourages us to listen to our bodies and enjoy the workout.

Ruth inspired me, along with thousands of others, to literally jump into a new dimension of fitness. Now, as the president of the Aquatic Exercise Association, I am continually reminded of the positive way that water exercise can influence lives. It has changed my life and through it I have developed friendships across the globe. Thanks, Ruth!

So follow the invitation—"Come on in, the water's great!"—and feel young at any age!

Julie See

PART
I

COME ON IN, THE WATER'S GREAT!

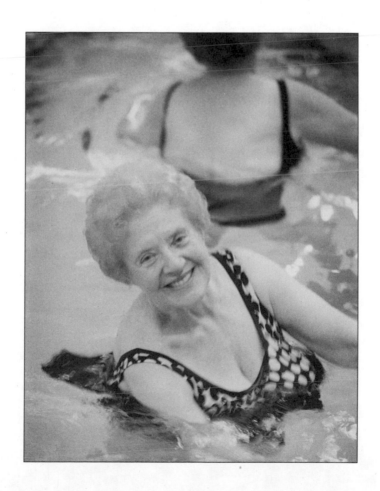

CHAPTER 1

THE BENEFITS OF WATER EXERCISE

I'm so glad that you're making this commitment to your health. You're certainly not alone. Every year 4 million people turn to water exercise. What makes water exercise so popular? It's wonderful and it works, it feels good to exercise in the water, and it's not a drudgery!

Compared to land exercise, water exercise is

- more fun and enjoyable,
- more effective and efficient, and
- more comfortable and safe.

Land exercise offers tremendous benefits, but too often those benefits are accompanied by aches and pains, overheating, sweating, and feelings of exhaustion. Water allows us to achieve all the wonderful benefits of exercise without experiencing these side effects. After water exercise, you'll feel refreshed and full of energy.

Exercising in the water helps eliminate feelings of self-consciousness because no one can see what you're doing. You don't have to fear that you won't succeed or that others will be watching you. If you're not quite sure that water exercise is for you, plunge into this chapter. I'll explain why millions of mature adults like you derive great physical benefits from exercising in water. If you're still not convinced, then I *challenge* you to use the exercises in this book and experience the benefits firsthand.

Why does water exercise work so well? There are many factors, but I think the major one is the buoyancy of the water.

With age, many people are unable to exercise in traditional ways due to minor changes in their bodies. At that point water exercise becomes ideal. The buoyancy of the water allows you to move around without getting hurt; you are able to work out with as much vigor as you want without the jarring impact associated with land exercise.

When you are submerged to shoulder depth in water, you experience an apparent weight loss of 90%. This means that if you weigh 150 pounds you will exercise at approximately 15 pounds. This apparent weight loss dramatically decreases the stress on the weight-bearing joints. This is why, for many people, water exercise is the safest fitness activity.

TOTAL FITNESS THROUGH WATER EXERCISE

Regular water exercise can improve all five components of physical fitness: aerobic fitness, muscle strength, muscle endurance, flexibility, and body composition. Each of these components plays a vital role in the body's health. You should try to be fit in as many of these ways as possible.

AEROBIC FITNESS

We all know that it's important for our heart, lungs, veins, and arteries to be healthy. The best way to achieve aerobic fitness is through aerobic exercise; aerobic exercise consists of at least 20 minutes of continuous activity that increases your heart rate to 65-85% of maximum (see pp. 23-26). To maintain aerobic fitness, you must engage in aerobic exercise activities at least three times a week.

Some people think that as they get older they will be unable to exercise as intensely or as long as they could when they were younger. Not true! In fact most of the decline in aerobic capacity that they attribute to age is actually caused by inactivity.

BETTY BALKS

Every time I saw Betty, a regular customer at the local breakfast/gossip restaurant, I'd stop to visit. The conversation always came around to her aching back and lack of energy.

I'd always invite Betty to one of my Aqua Challenge classes, and she'd always decline, saying she was afraid of the water, didn't like the water, didn't like being cold, and wouldn't wear a swimsuit until she lost 20 pounds. I countered all of those excuses, explaining that she wouldn't have to get her hair or even her face wet, she could hold on to the edge of the pool during the entire class, she'd be warm once she started moving, and that no one in the class had a perfect body. I told her she could cover up with a towel until she got to the pool and that no one would see her once she was in the water.

None of this made any difference to Betty. She continued to complain about her back and lack of energy, and I continued to praise water exercise.

One day Betty startled me by saying that she was thinking of coming to my class. One of her friends was in it. According to Betty, her friend was no swimmer or bathing beauty either, and she loved water exercise.

Sure enough, Betty showed up the next week. She came early, wore her towel to the edge of the pool, and got in before anyone could see her in her swimsuit. She stood in the shallowest part of the pool and hung on to the edge as I'd told her she could.

After five classes, Betty gave up wearing the towel, let go of the edge, and stood nearer to her friend. After eight classes, she had moved completely away from the edge of the pool and was visiting with everyone in class. After 12 classes (4 weeks), Betty started bringing other friends and morning breakfast buddies with her. And, finally, after 16 classes, Betty told me that her back hardly bothered her anymore.

Now when I see Betty at the local breakfast spot, she looks bright and fresh. She's the one singing the praises of water exercise, and I realize how I must sound when I get going! The benefits of water exercise are so far reaching that Betty and I can talk forever and not run out of good things to say about it.

She always tells her friends that I'm the one who gave her more energy and her new body. The truth is, I only gave Betty the means to improve herself, her outlook, and her health. Betty did all the work. She thinks I'm the best thing about class. I think she is. Even after 6 years.

What does this mean to you? It means you can exercise aerobically for as many years as you want, and you can work out as hard as you want. It means you can start exercising now and see dramatic improvements, even if you haven't exercised before!

Just what improvements can you expect from a good aerobic water exercise program? Three things: First, because you'll burn more calories, aerobic exercise will help you lose or control your weight. Second, it improves your respiratory (breathing) system so you don't develop shortness of breath. Third, it improves your circulatory system, keeping the blood moving easily to all parts of your body.

Besides these benefits, aerobic exercise can protect you from coronary heart disease. Regular aerobic exercise can reduce almost all risk factors of coronary disease (see Table 1.1) which can be changed.

Table 1.1

Primary Risk Factors For Coronary Heart Disease

These risk factors can be reduced through regular aerobic activity, such as water exercise.

Hypertension (high blood pressure)
High cholesterol and blood lipid levels
Smoking
Obesity
Atherosclerosis (hardening of the arteries)
Diabetes
Sedentary lifestyle (lack of physical activity)
Stress

MUSCLE STRENGTH

Lifting a box, moving furniture, and pulling—all these activities require certain muscles to exert force at one time. The more able you are to exert such force, the greater your muscle strength.

Most strengthening programs involve lifting weights; water provides resistance that acts like a weight. Since it's harder to walk through water than through air, it stands to reason that it's more work (moving against resistance) to walk through water. We can strengthen our muscles in the water, with or without equipment. The water's resistance, especially when combined with equipment, can make even simple movements challenging and provide a sufficient load to improve muscle strength.

Just moving through the water powerfully, you'll improve this second component of physical fitness. You'll be able to lift grandchildren and bags of groceries more easily. Better yet, you'll be able to get out of cars and chairs more easily!

MUSCLE ENDURANCE

You may not be interested in building muscles, but neither do you want your muscles to fatigue quickly. What you need is muscle endurance, the ability to repeat resistance activities many times. Muscle endurance is also called *tone*. Tone can be achieved sooner against the water's resistance than in workouts on land. Instead of the powerful movements used to build strength, steady movements through the water improve tone. Repeating any exercise 15 to 30 times will improve tone. If you're water walking, you need to walk longer. If you're doing kneelifts, you need to do more of them less forcefully. If you're exercising your arms, you need to repeat the exercise more times. If your exercise program is well planned, tone can be improved during your regular water exercise. Chapter 6 gives specific toning exercises.

Tone is something that can be maintained well into your older years. When you have it, you'll be able to stand up taller and longer, golf without an electric cart for 18 holes instead of 9, dance more than one dance at a wedding, and brush your teeth without your arm getting tired.

FLEXIBILITY

Flexibility is the ability of the joints to move through a normal range of motion. People who decide to exercise often ignore flexibility. Most of us just want to look good; we don't think flexibility will help us do that.

Flexibility, however, is important in everyday life. It's much easier to get dressed if you have good flexibility. You can reach across the table to set or clear it more easily if you are flexible. Flexibility helps you reach for the seatbelt. Flexibility may protect you from injury. During a fall, the joints are usually hyperextended, or pushed beyond their normal range. If you're flexible, your joints may be able to tolerate a momentary hyperextension without injury. If you're inflexible, your joints will not be able to tolerate it, and injury can occur.

So flexibility *is* important both in everyday life and in special circumstances. Think about how much more simple flexibility makes it to bend over to tie your shoes, to cross your legs to tie your shoes, to reach out from bed to turn on the light, to wash your hair, and best of all to hug a child.

To gain flexibility you need to stretch each muscle for 30 to 60 seconds. Because of the lessened effect of gravity in the water, joints may be moved through a greater range of motion and stretched more effectively without increasing pressure. Water lets you stretch in ways that may not be possible on land. All of the joints that are underwater will feel relaxed and, usually, pain-free.

Although flexibility does tend to decrease with age, arthritis, other chronic disease, or injuries can also affect it. Flexibility is an example of the "move it or lose it" concept. If your joints are not used through their normal range of motion on a regular basis, they eventually lose a part of that range. Moving your arms, legs, and torso as far as easily possible in all directions can slow or avoid loss of flexibility.

Maintaining flexibility is important for bending over to retrieve something you've dropped, reaching up to the top shelf in your closet, reaching behind your head to fix your hair, and catching yourself if you slip on the ice. Chapter 6 includes specific stretching exercises to improve and maintain flexibility.

BODY COMPOSITION

Body composition is the proportion of fat body mass to lean body mass. Most of us need to work toward less fat body mass and more lean body mass. Body weight is not as important as body composition. As we age, we tend to lose some of our lean body mass; if we continue to weigh the same, lean body mass has been replaced by fat body mass. The scales can't tell us if we have good body composition.

The average person burns 450 to 700 calories while exercising for 1 hour. In the water, 77% of the calories burned come from stored fat, helping to reduce fat mass.

ADDITIONAL BENEFITS

That's it! A good water workout will help you be fit in all five major physical fitness components. But what about other qualities we want to improve?

MINOR FITNESS COMPONENTS

The minor components of physical fitness include speed, power, agility, reaction time, coordination, and balance. Each of these decreases with age. As with all other "aging-process" deteriorations, these can be maintained or reversed with regular water exercise.

Reaction time usually slows with age, but doesn't have to. By exercising three times a week for 20 minutes, older adults can have the same reaction times as college-aged women.

Coordination and balance are especially important as we age. Loss of coordination and balance contributes to falls which are a serious health problem for older adults. Working against the water's resistance and in a different medium definitely improves coordination and balance.

SKELETAL BENEFITS

The skeletal benefits of water exercise are only recently being studied. The findings are impressive.

Osteoporosis, a condition in which the bones gradually lose some of the minerals (including calcium) that make them strong and become fragile and more likely to cause pain or break (see p. 107), is an example of a problem that can be mitigated by diet and exercise. Osteoporosis affects women more often than men; white, small-boned, postmenopausal women are at the highest risk. It can eventually lead to deformity, disability, and severe physical and emotional pain. Eating a diet rich in calcium and phosphorus and moderate, regular, vigorous exercise will retard, and sometimes reverse, osteoporosis. It used to be thought that the exercise had to be weight bearing and impact producing (walking, running, aerobic dancing) to have a beneficial effect on the bones. Now we know that stress on the place in the bone where new bone cells form is what triggers an increase in bone density.

Forcefully pushing and pulling your arms and legs through the water's resistance can assist in building or maintaining bone density as well as muscle mass.

PSYCHOLOGICAL BENEFITS

The mind-body connection is another excellent reason to exercise. Exercise improves our emotional well being, outlook, enjoyment of life, and self-esteem. The emotionally stable person with a positive attitude will be less likely to suffer from physical diseases, pain, and immune system deficiencies. The mind-body connection also correlates with mental sharpness, alertness, and intelligence. Those who work out regularly test better in complex decision making, according to researcher and author T. Young.

YOU'RE GETTING BETTER

As wonderful as these benefits are, I've saved the best for last. Many so-called effects of aging are not inevitable. In fact, The American Medical Association's Committee on Aging found that it is almost impossible to distinguish between the effects of aging and the effects of inactivity. Researchers G. Van Camp and B. Boyer believe that the real effects of aging don't occur during our current life span, even postulating a human life span of 280 years!

The key to aging gracefully is activity, both mental and physical. The often-heard phrase "use it or lose it" definitely applies. As Kenny Moore, former Olympic marathon runner, said, "You don't stop exercising because you grow old. You grow old because you stop exercising."

In his book *Creative Aging* Dr. W. M. Bortz says, "There's a difference between biological and chronological age. Some people, eighty years old by the calendar, have body tissue with the vitality of a thirty year old."

One last quote, from The American Medical Association: "Routine exercise helps reduce the risk of a host of degenerative and chronic diseases, including coronary heart disease, diabetes, obesity and osteoporosis."

I've found this information to be so motivating! It tells us it's not chronological age that makes us look and feel old, it's inactivity. If we're active, we can look and feel our best. And water is the near-perfect medium in which to be active.

The following list of problems, although not limited to older adults, are generally associated with aging.

Arthritis	High blood sugar
Back problems	High cholesterol
Chronic pain	Insomnia
Constipation	Low energy
Decreased lung capacity	Obesity
Decreased range of motion	Osteoporosis
Depression	Poor muscle strength
Diabetes	Senility
Heart conditions	Stiffness
High blood pressure	Stress and tension

If you think this list represents the inevitable health problems of age, you're wrong! Many of these conditions are directly related to inactive lifestyle.

Our bodies are made to move and to be used. If they aren't used, they deteriorate. That's why we see some 80 year olds with 30-year-old body tissue and some 30 year olds with 80-year-old body tissue. But biological age needn't correlate to chronological age. We are fortunate to be able to keep our biological age low through something as simple, effective, and enjoyable as water exercise.

ARTHRITIS SUBMERGED

Let me tell you about someone who wasn't reluctant to come to class. Barb wanted to exercise, but her arthritis was so bad that she had trouble dressing, moving around the house, and making it through the day. As soon as her doctor recommended water exercise, Barb joined us. She had trouble at first because the water wasn't as warm as most of us would have liked. If she didn't keep moving, she became chilled and she'd ache even more. She said it felt like that horrible, damp ache many of us feel in cold, rainy weather.

I did some research, and within a week we had Barb wearing a full unitard (like a swimsuit that goes to the ankle and wrists), webbed water exercise gloves, and a Wet Wrap vest to keep her warm and shoes to help cushion any impact.

She also did a longer warm-up, and kept her movements small at first. She did a fairly short cool-down, so she'd still be warm and toasty when she got out of the pool. The changes worked! We were so thrilled! Barb was able to exercise safely without causing herself more pain.

And as she continued to work out with our class, she experienced more benefits. She was able to dress more easily, to reach farther in more directions, and to get around the house with fewer problems. She had less pain, felt more comfortable even in the morning, and she started getting out and around town. Yes, Barb still has arthritis, but she feels and looks good now because she stands taller. The doctor who sent her to class is overwhelmed by her progress. He just keeps saying, "Whatever you're doing, keep doing it." And she does.

People who continue to exercise are less likely to experience "age-related" health problems. Regular water exercise can

- decrease arthritis pain,
- decrease back pain,
- lessen chronic pain,
- improve regularity,
- increase lung capacity,
- improve flexibility,
- improve the outlook on life,
- regulate blood-sugar levels,
- improve heart functions,
- control blood pressure,
- regulate cholesterol,
- maintain good sleep patterns,
- increase energy,
- help maintain safe body composition,
- maintain bone density,
- improve muscle strength and tone,
- improve some mental functions,
- decrease anger, anxiety, and impulsiveness,
- improve the quality of life, and even
- improve sexual interest and satisfaction.

Water exercise is excellent for older adults, even those who have not been active for years. The benefits tend to intensify with age.

Older adults who have been out of condition for a long time can increase fitness levels with minimal risk of injury using water exercise. As I mentioned, a body loses approximately 90% of its weight in shoulder-depth water. The soothing pressure of the water lessens joint swelling and pain and increases flexibility and mobility. Water provides a soft, easy workout or a hard, energetic workout, depending on the force of the movement used.

The benefits of water exercise are tremendous. I'm sold on it because I've experienced those benefits—as a water exerciser and instructor of thousands of mature adults. I hope that you're sold on it too. Let's get ready for the water!

CHAPTER 2

BEFORE YOU GET IN THE POOL

Before you begin a class or start your own program, you should either take a fitness-assessment test or see your doctor to determine your beginning exercise level.

FITNESS TESTING AND HEALTH HISTORIES

If you sign up for a class, you will probably be asked to fill out and sign various forms.

One form is called an informed consent, a disclaimer, or a release. This form does not ask you to sign away your rights. It just reminds you that there are risks associated with the exercise program you will be participating in. If you sign the form, you will be saying that you understand those risks, you accept them. A sample form is included here (see Table 2.1).

Table 2.1

Sample Release Form

REPRESENTATION, RELEASE AND AGREEMENT

PLEASE READ CAREFULLY AND SIGN BELOW. "I, fully understanding that the programs and exercises of THE FITNESS FIRM require vigorous physical activity, hereby represent and acknowledge that my physical condition permits me to participate in THE FITNESS FIRM programs and exercises. I further acknowledge that I have been advised that at any time I am having physical difficulty, I will immediately inform the Class Teacher and will be automatically excused from classes. I have volunteered to participate in this program and accept the responsibility. I understand that the possibility of exercise injuries or disorders does exist. I acknowledge and accept those risks.

I further realize that I will not be accepted for participation in the program if THE FITNESS FIRM knows of any reason why my participation would be dangerous to my health.

I also release and discharge on behalf of myself, my heirs, assigns and successor in interest, all officers, directors, agents, and employees and other representatives of THE FITNESS FIRM and its insurers, from any and all claim, damages, demands, and liabilities arising out of or in any way related to participation in THE FITNESS FIRM activities and the use of any of its exercises, procedures or other results attained therefrom."

MEMBER'S SIGNATURE	DATE

Another form you usually have to fill out is called a health history, a general history questionnaire, or a student profile form. This form commonly asks information such as your name, address, and emergency information (a contact person's name and phone number). You are usually asked to provide a physician's name, phone number, and address as well. Medical information about possible risk factors you may have for heart disease is usually included on this form. Other questions regarding your medical history and your current fitness level are also asked. It is important you fill this form out completely and honestly so that the instructor is able to make special modifications for your program, if necessary.

After reviewing the health history form, many organizations require fitness testing. Most fitness tests are brief and allow the instructor to modify a program for your individual needs.

If you have a history of heart disease, hypertension, or chronic illness, or maybe you're simply over 40 (and most of the world is!), you may be asked to have your doctor sign a medical clearance form. The instructor uses the form (see Table 2.2) to gain further information regarding your participation in class. It generally tells what type of activity you'll be involved in, how often you'll exercise, how long you'll exercise each time, and the intensity level of the class. It asks if there are any types of movements that you should avoid or any possible restrictions to your exercise regime. Your doctor has to sign and date the form and return it to the instructor before you participate in class.

The last form you'll probably see just prior to beginning class is often called a "class policy." This is an information sheet that tells you the rules regarding the pool, where to change, if it is safe to leave valuables in the locker room, and so forth.

But I'm On My Own

If you're going to create your own program, you should decide what you'd like to do and then tell your physician. It is especially important to check with your physician if you have, or ever had

- advice from a physician not to exercise,
- arteriosclerosis (hardening of the arteries),
- arthritis or other joint problems,
- asthma or other allergies,
- chronic illness,
- diabetes,
- difficulty with physical exercise (dizziness, breathlessness, recent surgery, anxiety, or depression),
- excessive stress,
- high blood lipids and cholesterol level,
- a history of lung problems,

- hypertension (high blood pressure),
- individual or family history of heart disease,
- muscle, joint, or back disorders,
- obesity, or
- smoking habits.

Remember that water exercise can be an exertive program. Your physician should know of your intention to participate.

OTHER THINGS TO CONSIDER

While formal fitness testing may be done at the fitness or health club, you can get a feel for your fitness level before attending classes or beginning your own workout.

Go for a 15 or 20 minute water walk at a comfortable pace. If you feel winded or exhausted afterward, you probably need to begin more slowly than traditional water aerobics class in a health club. Start by walking 5 minutes a day. When you're comfortable with that, increase the time to 10 minutes a day. Work up to water walking for 15 to 20 minutes without exhaustion. At that point you'll be ready to advance to basic water exercise.

If you aren't winded after 20 minutes but your legs feel totally exhausted, begin with water toning before starting a complete water exercise program. Water toning strengthens the muscles in your legs and arms so you can keep moving for a longer period of time without exhausting your muscles.

You'll find walking and toning programs in chapters 4 and 6, respectively. Do a little of the program you choose each day.

Here's a simple flexibility test: Reach up as high as you can on your kitchen cupboards. If your arms won't extend all the way up, it's time to start water exercise. Can you bend over and touch your toes from either a standing or sitting position? If you can't touch, it's time for water exercise to help you increase the flexibility in those joints.

It's not necessary to be fit before beginning water exercise. Don't worry if you aren't flexible. That will come during your workouts. Don't get discouraged. After you've been in the water for a few weeks, you'll see improvement.

Table 2.2

Sample Medical Clearance Form

SUZY INSTRUCTOR
123 MAIN STREET   ANYTOWN, USA
443-127-5858

Your patient, _____, has applied to participate in an
aquatic exercise program. The class meets three times a week for one hour and
involves aerobics using all major muscle groups. It is moderate in intensity and
light impact.

Please list any medications that your patient is currently taking and how they will
affect the heart rate response (elevate, depress or no change).
MEDICATION AND EFFECT ON EXERCISE HEART RATE

Please list any restrictions, modifications or recommendations for your patient's
exercise program.

_____

_____

_____

_____

Please list any special concerns you may have regarding this patient (i.e.,
arrhythmia, low back problems, arthritis, etc.).

_____

_____

_____

_____

Please list the target heart rate, rate of perceived exertion or general exercise
intensity at which this patient should exercise.

_____

Sincerely,

Suzy Instructor

My patient, _____, has my approval to enroll in an
aquatic exercise program at _____ (facility name) with
the above restrictions, modifications and recommendations.
PHYSICIAN'S SIGNATURE _____

SAFETY FIRST

Here are some tips to keep the program you're taking or creating safe:

• Always warm up for at least 10 minutes before beginning your program, even if you are pressed for time or arrive late to class. The warm-up prepares your muscles for exercise.

• Exercise at a level you can maintain for most of the workout. Walk or move slowly if you tire, but do not stop completely until after you cool down.

• You know your body best; listen to it. Don't panic if the following occur, but do stop vigorous exercise, move slowly, and notify your exercise partner, instructor, and/or doctor if you experience any of these warning signals:

  – Abnormal heart beat

  – Pain or pressure in the chest, arm, or throat

  – Nausea

  – Extreme weakness

  – Excessive fatigue

  – Dizziness, cold sweat, pallor, blueness, or near fainting

  – Flare up of arthritis

  – Breathlessness

  – Shinsplints, sidestitch, or charley horse.

• If you must cut your workout short on busy days, cool down before you leave the water. This will protect you from a lightheaded feeling.

• Wait 1 hour after a light meal or 2 hours after a heavy meal before exercising.

• Do not drink alcoholic beverages before exercising. Alcohol impairs balance and coordination.

• Work out for fun and aerobic fitness, not for perfection or performance. This is a noncompetitive activity. Individual styles are encouraged.

• Keep your mouth clear of food and other objects during exercise.

• No pain should increase while participating in water exercise. If you experience increased pain, stop exercising and notify your exercise partner, instructor, and/or doctor.

• Drink 8 ounces of water before exercising, 8 ounces during exercise, and 8 ounces after exercise. You can usually keep a soft plastic water container at the pool edge. It's important to keep your body hydrated; we don't realize how much we sweat in the pool since the water washes it away.

• Be comfortable enough in the water to right yourself if you slip and fall forward or backward under the water. It's not necessary to swim well, but you should be able to save your life by getting to the edge of the pool if necessary.

• Know what to do in an emergency. Know where the phone is, how to use it, and what emergency number to use.

• Know where the first aid equipment is.

• Know where the fire exit is located from the locker room, pool area, and hallway.

• Know how to evacuate the locker room, pool area, and hallway in case of a tornado or civil defense warning.

WHAT DO I DO?

The American College of Sports Medicine has set up specific guidelines for aerobic workouts based on frequency (how often the training occurs), intensity (how hard the workout is), type (the kind of training), and time (how long the workout lasts).

• Frequency should be at least three, but usually no more than five, times a week. There should be no more than 2 days between workouts. Beginners should try to exercise three times a week with a day off between each workout (see Table 2.3).

• Intensity should be in the target range for heart rate or in the "somewhat hard" to "heavy" range in perceived exertion.

Table 2.3

Sample Calendar

Sun.	Mon.	Tues.	Wed.	Thurs.	Fri.	Sat.
	1	2	3	4	5	6
7	8	9	10	11	12	13
14	15	16	17	18	19	20
21	22	23	24	25	26	27
28	29	30				

• Type has to be continuous (with no stops) and rhythmical and use the large muscles. The large muscles include the front and back of the thighs and the buttocks. It is fine to use other muscles, but they won't burn as many calories as the large muscles. Since leg exercise is more energy and calorie consuming than arm exercise, you should always keep your legs moving.

• Time should be 20 to 60 minutes of continuous exercise. Beginners should work toward at least 20 minutes. As your body adapts, you can increase the length of your workout.

If your program meets these four qualifications, you will be assured a good aerobic, calorie-consuming workout.

WORKOUT INTENSITY

Make sure that you exercise hard enough to challenge yourself. Get to the "huff and puff" stage. You have to breathe faster and deeper than normal in order to achieve aerobic fitness.

If you're following your own program, you should evaluate how hard you're working about three times during each workout. In a class, the instructor will ask you to monitor your workout intensity. I'll review information about heart rates and alternative intensity evaluations (including overexertion) in this section so you become familiar with the basics.

HEART RATES

Heart rate monitoring provides a way to assess the intensity or exertion level of a workout. It will show if you are not exercising hard enough, exercising hard enough to achieve benefits, or exercising too hard. There are several different terms used when discussing heart rates: resting heart rate, working heart-rate range, minimum working heart rate, maximum working heart rate, and recovery heart rate. Table 2.4 shows the ranges and averages for these rates.

Resting Heart Rate. The resting heart rate is the number of heart beats per minute when the body is at rest. This count is usually taken for 1 minute before getting out of bed in the morning or after lying down for 30 minutes. You'll get a more accurate resting heart rate count if you take it on three separate occasions and average the numbers.

Usually as fitness levels increase, resting heart rate decreases. The average resting heart rate is about 72 beats per minute. Medications affect that number. People with hypertension and people who ingest large amounts of caffeine or nicotine have different resting heart rates.

Working Heart-Rate Range. The working heart-rate range is also called the target zone. It's the range you need to work within to increase calorie consumption and aerobic conditioning.

Minimum Working Heart Rate. The minimum working heart rate is the low end of the range. It is the lowest number of heart beats per minute required for conditioning.

Table 2.4

Heart Rates and Averages	
	Heart Rates (bpm)

Average	155
Maximum	150
	145
	140
	135
	130
Average	125
Working	120
Range	115
	110
	105
	100
	95
Average	90
Minimum	85
	80
Average Recovery	75
	70
Average	65
Resting	60

Maximum Working Heart Rate. The maximum working heart rate is the high end of the range. It is the highest number of heart beats per minute desirable during exercise. *Working at the maximum can be dangerous.* It's best to work at the midpoint of the target zone.

Recovery Heart Rate. The recovery heart rate measures how quickly your cardiorespiratory system recovers from exercise. Usually a well-conditioned person recovers faster than an unconditioned person. In other words, 5 minutes after the cool-down, a well-conditioned person's heart beats per minute will be lower than an unconditioned person's.

Using Heart Rates

Heart rates are usually checked for 6 seconds and then converted to a 1-minute rate by adding a zero (multiplying by 10) to the 6-second number.

Some exercisers check the carotid artery (along the windpipe in the throat), while others prefer to test the radial pulse (at the wrist). When counting the pulse at either place, remember to use your index and middle fingers with very light pressure only. Heavy pressure to the carotid could restrict blood supply to the brain. The thumb shouldn't be used since it has a pulse of its

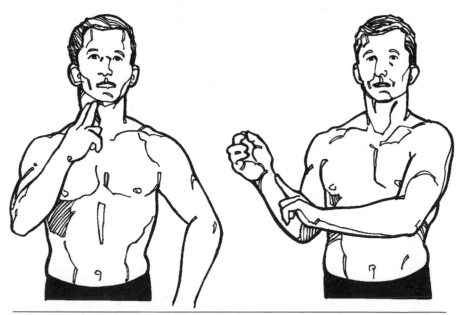

Checking heart rates at the cartoid artery (left) and the radial pulse (right).

own. If you have difficulty finding pulses at either of these places, try putting your hand over your heart and counting the beats.

Heart rates are generally lower during water exercise than during land exercise. There are several theories to explain this. It is thought that since the water cools the body, the heart doesn't have to beat as hard. Also, because water lessens the effect of gravity and compresses (provides some support), the heart doesn't have to beat as hard.

The Aquatic Exercise Association's heart rate chart (see Table 2.5) takes into account a lower working heart rate in the water.

ALTERNATIVE INTENSITY EVALUATIONS

A study done by the American College of Sports Medicine showed that we're very good at sensing our own intensity levels. If you are unable to check your pulse during exercise, you can use the "rate of perceived exertion" (see Table 2.6). While looking at the chart and exercising, estimate the exertion level of your workout. If it falls in the "somewhat hard" to "heavy" category, you will be in the target zone (within minimum to maximum range) for the chart. "Light" exertion may not be enough for conditioning to occur. If you feel that you are moving into the "very heavy" area, you should cut back, since that could be dangerously high.

Table 2.5

Aquatic Exercise Association Aquatics Heart Rate Chart

Age	Min. Working Heart Rate	Max. Working Heart Rate
20-29	124	179
30-39	119	161
40-49	114	152
50-59	108	143
60-69	103	134
70+	98	125

It is important to avoid the overexertion that working at a high intensity could cause. The signs of overexertion are

- breathlessness,
- dizziness,
- extreme fatigue,
- nausea,
- a red face, and
- a very high heart rate (over the target zone).

If any of these symptoms occur, walk slowly to recover and work out at a lower intensity next time.

PRINCIPLES OF FITNESS

Let's review some basic principles of physical fitness. These are overload, progressive overload, adaptation, specificity, reversibility, and variability.

Table 2.6

American College of Sports Medicine Rate of Perceived Exertion Chart	
0	nothing
0.5	very, very light (just noticeable)
1.0	very light
2	light (weak)
3	moderate
4 } Target zone	somewhat hard
5	heavy (strong)
6	
7	very heavy
8	
9	
10	very, very heavy (almost max.)

OVERLOAD

Overload means that to improve, you need to do more than you are used to doing. If you normally walk 1/2 mile three times a week, you can improve your fitness level by walking four times a week, by going faster, or by increasing the distance.

PROGRESSIVE OVERLOAD

Progressive overload means to gradually increase the demands on your body. To go from inactivity to walking briskly for 1 mile would be increasing the load too quickly for most people. It is better to make smaller changes and add on gradually.

ADAPTATION

Adaptation means that your body will adapt to the changes you make. For example, if you walk 1 mile three times a week, your body will eventually become strong enough that you can either walk farther in the same length of time or walk the mile more quickly. Adaptation is the change in your body as you exercise.

SPECIFICITY

Specificity says that whatever you specifically work on will improve. If you walk and never stretch, your legs will become stronger and your cardiorespiratory system will improve, but you will not necessarily increase your flexibility. If you do only upper body work, the lower body will not develop. It is important to work on each of the major components of physical fitness that you want to improve.

REVERSIBILITY

Reversibility means "use it or lose it." It takes approximately 8 weeks for the body to start improving from exercise, but only 2 weeks of no exercise will cause a decrease in fitness levels! Fitness cannot be stored. Because of reversibility, it is important to choose exercise you enjoy and look forward to. Any type of vigorous exercise will work, but it will only work if you continue to do it. Water exercise is fun because the water is enjoyable and because the other participants in the program make it a constantly changing experience. Best of all, it is extremely effective.

VARIABILITY

Variability means that, if possible, you should change the type of exercise you do to continue improving. If you've been doing water walking for 3 or 4 months, try a water toning class, a water aerobics class, or a deep-water workout. These programs are described in chapter 4.

WHERE DO I GO?

So, you're interested and wondering where you can find a water exercise class. Look in the yellow pages under

- exercise and physical fitness programs,
- gymnasiums,
- health and fitness program consultants,
- health clubs,
- swimming instruction,
- swimming pools—private,
- swimming pools—public,
- toning salons, and
- weight control services.

Check the newspaper. Call the local YMCA, YWCA, community center, or recreation department. If they don't have exactly the program you want, give the class they're offering a try. You may be able to participate in most of the class and add other exercises you want to do.

If the classes offered do not meet your needs, you can create your own program. You won't need to rent a pool if you decide to exercise in the water alone. If you don't have access to a private pool, you can sign up at most pool clubs to attend during open swim or lap swim times. Find your own special part or lane of the pool, and do your exercise program there.

It may feel a little intimidating at first to be the only one whose feet are touching bottom, but water exercise is so enjoyable that other people will probably want to join in. If you like music, a company called Hydrophonics makes a water-proof cassette player. You can exercise to your favorite music or try one of the aquatic fitness program tapes available from the Aquatic Exercise Association and other groups. Information on Hydrophonics and the Aquatic Exercise Association is located in the appendix.

WHAT DO I WEAR?

While most of us may be convinced that water exercise will be good for us, very few of us are sure that we want to be seen in our swimsuits. If you're comfortable with your swimsuit, that's what you should wear. If you're not comfortable with it, there are several alternatives available.

Fitness and swim clothing manufacturers are making special clothing for water exercise. You may want to wear knee-length shorts or calf- or ankle-length tights under your regular swimsuit. Some women prefer tights or shorts with a sports bra and leotard; others wear a unitard which can be worn alone or with a swimsuit or leotard over it. Men usually wear

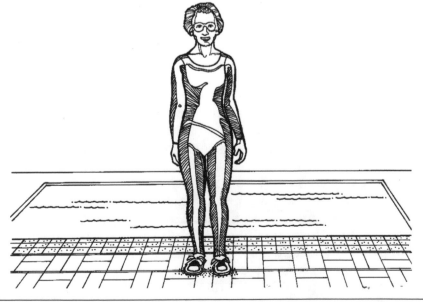

Wearing a unitard can keep you warmer in the water.

either their swim shorts or knee-length shorts. The full unitard, sometimes bought as a "wetskin," is recommended for people with arthritis because it offers additional warmth.

WHAT ELSE DO I NEED?

Now that we've discussed the basics, what else might be needed? I feel that it's very important to wear water exercise shoes. The shoes protect your feet in the locker room, on the pool deck, and in the water. They protect you from slipping on a rough pool bottom and give you more cushion during the light impact that you'll experience.

There are different types of shoes for different purposes. If you'll be participating in a program with jumping and jogging, you need a shoe that fits snugly and has some cushioning. If your program is mostly walking or toning in place, the shoe doesn't need as much cushioning.

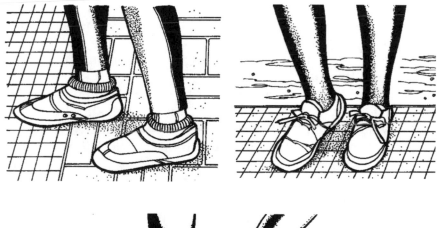

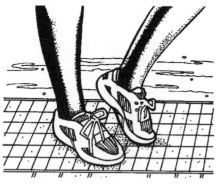

Water shoes with a good, snug fit will protect your feet in and around the pool.

A word of caution about choosing shoes. They should be comfortable, but tight. If they're too loose, water dragging against them will pull them off your feet. Make sure they're snug; they should feel almost too tight. Be aware that wet laces can be hard to untie, especially if there is arthritis in the fingers. Most aqua shoes are slip-on or have slides on the laces.

Many students like to wear bathing or shower caps to protect their hair. This is okay as long as you're not feeling warm. During exercise, your body generates heat. That heat needs to be dissipated or it could be dangerous. Since most body heat is lost from the top of the head, it is unwise to wear a swim or shower cap when you're feeling hot and flushed. If yours is a moderate intensity program, you may not have a problem.

There's a plethora of water exercise equipment on the market. I am often asked which type of equipment is best. That is impossible to answer because the equipment is different, you are all different, and your purposes in using the equipment are different.

Having said that, I think the first type of equipment that can be added safely is webbed gloves. These gloves shouldn't give you any additional joint problems and they add resistance to make your workout more fun and more challenging.

The next addition would be buoyant or resistant dumbbells for upper body work. For lower body work, buoyant or resistant ankle cuffs make your workout more challenging.

If you decide to try equipment, be sure to follow the manufacturer's guidelines.

If you want to try equipment but can't find any in your area, check the appendix for catalog sources.

PART
II
WATER EXERCISES

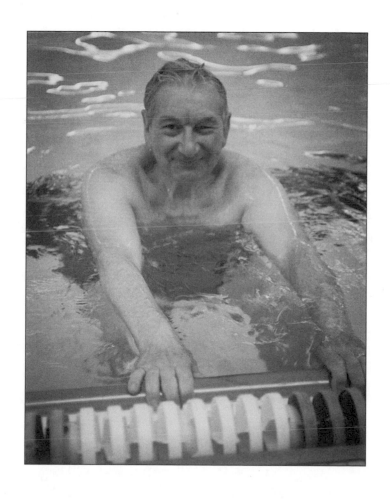

CHAPTER

3

THE WARM-UP

It's important to warm up before you exercise. In this chapter, I'll explain the why and how of warming up.

Warming up before exercising protects you from injury. Skipping the warm-up could result in muscle tears, joint damage, and cardiac problems, none of which is fun. Luckily, by warming up, you can avoid these unpleasant results. The warm-up prepares your muscles, joints, heart, and respiratory system for the workout that's coming.

It's important to go through at least 10 minutes (and preferably 15) of warm-up every time you exercise, even if you feel rushed. At the end of the warm-up, your body should feel warmer thermally than it was when you started. You should be breathing deeper and more frequently. Remember, failing to warm up can lead to injuries.

A full warm-up consists of three portions: a thermal warm-up that starts your muscles moving and begins lubricating your joints, a prestretch that prevents injury in the workout to come, and an aerobic warm-up that safely increases your heart rate.

THERMAL WARM-UP

The thermal warm-up consists of moving your arms, bending your knees and elbows, moving your legs, and moving around through the water. It's also called a musculoskeletal warm-up because at this point you don't care if the heart starts to beat faster or not. You just need to warm the muscles and lubricate the joints.

Remember to move your arms. The movements should begin small, eventually getting larger. For example, begin with a small forward armlift, eventually lifting your arm forward as high as you can.

Here's a sample thermal warm-up you can do each session. Do each exercise for 30 seconds.

*T*he thermal warm-up should be done every time you exercise. It should last 3 to 5 minutes. *Never begin your exercise program without the thermal warm-up.*

Walk
Begin by walking forward and backward through the pool. Walk at least 10 steps forward, then back up 10 steps. Keep your body upright and your posture strong.

Long-stride walking
Continue walking, but lengthen your stride a little and start to swing your arms forward and backward as you walk. See Exercise 38.

Bent-knee walking
Continue walking, but crouch down as low as you can and walk with your knees bent, like Groucho Marx. Keep your torso upright. See Exercise 4.

Tiptoe walking
Now straighten up and walk forward and backward on tiptoe. Get up as high as you can, lift your ribs up, and stand as tall as possible. See Exercise 58.

Heel walking

This is difficult to do, but it's excellent for coordination and balance. Try to walk forward and backward on your heels. See Exercise 21.

Walk and roll

Now walk forward and backward, rolling heel to toe and taking strides as long as possible. See Exercises 66 and 67.

Side step

Side step one way through the water several times and then change direction. As you step to the side, lift your arms in front of you to the top of the water. As your feet step together, push your arms down in front of you. See Exercise 53.

Side step with a dip

Continue sideways walking but crouch down and get your shoulders wet as you step apart. Come up on tiptoe as your feet step together. See Exercise 55.

Low side step

Continue sideways walking, but stay in a crouch. Keep your shoulders wet, stay low in the water, and walk sideways, first in one direction and then in the other. See Exercise 39.

Shoulder rolls

Shoulder rolls get the muscles and the connective tissues in the joint ready for a more intense workout. Begin with small movements. Press your shoulders forward, then lift them up, then press them back, and then return to the beginning position. Later in the warm-up, after the joint has been used easily, you might want to do shoulder rolls with elbows out. This will increase the work on the shoulder joint. See Exercise 48.

PRESTRETCH

Prestretch is the next portion of the warm-up. Muscles that are tight from everyday living need to be stretched before they can safely work at high-intensity, full-range-of-motion capacity. It used to be thought that you could stretch first and then warm up. We now know that stretching does not effectively prevent injury if the muscles and joints aren't warmed up first.

You should never stretch cold muscles. If you're feeling shivery or cold in the water after the thermal warm-up, keep moving. Don't stretch yet. Increase the intensity of your movements and continue the warm-up exercises. Do not stretch until your muscles feel warm. If you begin to stretch and your muscle feels tight and does not stretch easily, your body is still too cool.

Frequently when I do the prestretch after the thermal warm-up, I start out warm and begin to cool off. To keep my body temperature up I walk, bounce, or jog between the stretches. This allows me to do all the stretching I need without the danger of stretching cold muscles.

There's another important thing to know about stretching. Stretches should be held, not bounced. When I was in school, we were taught to bounce while stretching. But bouncing while stretching actually causes microscopic muscle tears. Those tears make you less limber and tighten up your muscles more. In other words, bouncing during the stretch will cause exactly the opposite of the effect you're trying to achieve.

The safest way to stretch is to stretch and hold without moving. Move into the stretch, feel some tightness but no pain, and hold that position for 5 to 10 seconds. This may sound short, but it *is* adequate. Include the prestretches described and illustrated in every warm-up. Remember, hold them without bouncing!

Here are the stretch descriptions. Hold each stretch steadily for 5 to 10 seconds.

*R*emember not to bounce. These stretches should not hurt. Stay warm while stretching.

Calf stretch
See Exercise 7.

Calves are tight from walking, moving, and simply being in shoes with a high heel. Stand facing the edge of the pool. Hold on to the gutter and bring the toes of one foot up close to the pool wall. Step your other foot back as far as you can. Press the heel of your back foot down while leaning your torso forward over your hands. You should feel a stretch in the calf muscle of your back leg. If you don't feel a stretch, keep one foot close to the pool wall, and step your other foot back about 12 inches. Pull the toes of your back foot up as high as you can. At this point, you should feel a stretch in the calf of the back leg.

An alternative to this stretch, if those positions aren't comfortable or you don't feel the stretch, is to put the toes of your front foot up on the pool wall. This stretches the calf of your front leg.

Hip flexor stretch
See Exercise 26.

The hip flexor muscle, also called the iliopsoas, runs down the front of the inner thigh. It's very tight from daily sitting, walking, and general movement.

Stand facing the pool edge, hands on the gutter, and one foot close to the pool wall. Step your other foot back about 1-1/2 feet. Swing your hips forward and hold them there as hard as you can. This position is called a pelvic tilt. The knee of your back leg should point at the bottom of the pool; your heel should be up. The hip of your back leg should be pushing forward very hard. You should feel a stretch that starts about halfway down your inner thigh and moves up toward your stomach. That's the hip flexor muscle. If you don't feel a stretch in that position, here's another option.

Stand facing the pool edge with one hand on the pool edge. Your feet should be about 6 inches from the pool wall. Lift the heel of one leg up behind your body. If you can, grab your foot or ankle to hold it up. With your knee back just a little, go into the pelvic tilt position. In order to feel the stretch, your knee should be back just a little bit instead of pointing straight down, and your hip pushed forward.

Hamstring stretch
See Exercises 17 and 18.

The hamstring muscles are located in the back of the thigh. If you sit a lot, these muscles are usually tight.

Stand sideways to the pool edge. Put one hand on the gutter, and pull the knee of the leg that's away from the pool wall toward your chest. Hold your hand on the back of your thigh or under your knee. In that position, straighten your knee. You should feel easy tension in the back of the thigh. If you don't feel the tension, lower your leg a little and straighten your knee again.

If that position doesn't work for you, take a step away from the pool wall and face it. Put one foot up against the pool wall and lean over that leg. You can hold onto the leg that's against the pool wall for balance. As you lean forward over your leg, you should feel easy tension in the back of your thigh.

Pectoral stretch
See Exercises 42 and 43.

The pectoral, or chest, muscles are also tight from everyday living because we use our arms mostly in front of us.

Stand in chest-deep water. Interlace your fingers behind your back. While keeping your shoulders back, lift your arms as high as you can behind your back. This is an excellent stretch not only for your chest muscles but also for your shoulders. If this position isn't comfortable, try this.

Take your hands out of the water and interlace your fingers behind your head. Point both elbows out and back a little. You should feel your rib cage opening. In this position, you should feel a good stretch across your chest.

Aerobic Warm-Up

The final portion is called the aerobic warm-up. The aerobic warm-up is very important because you need to gradually increase the load on your heart and lungs. If the increase is too rapid, it could stress the heart. This part of the warm-up is actually the beginning of the aerobic phase. You move straight from the aerobic warm-up into low-intensity aerobics. You will gradually get your heart beating a little bit faster and your lungs working a little bit more, using your lung capacity more quickly. Your respiration rate (how often you breathe each minute) will increase. As long as you're not out of breath by the end of this portion, the aerobic warm-up is probably doing the job. You should be huffing and puffing a little.

The aerobic warm-up begins with jogging moves and gradually progresses to jogging more quickly or jogging with more power. Here's an example of a good aerobic warm-up. Each exercise should be done for 30 seconds.

*I*n general your knees will be safe throughout your exercise program if you remember not to lock them, twist them, or move them too quickly.

- Locking means overstraightening the knee.

- Twisting occurs when your feet are planted on the pool bottom and your knees point in a different direction than your toes. The knee and toes of the same leg should always point in the same direction.

- Moving the knees too quickly can happen if you try to move at "land speed" when exercising in the water. Keep your movements slow and controlled.

Jog
Jog forward 8 to 16 jogs (depending on the length of the pool) and backward the same number.

High knee jog
Jog forward and backward with your knees high, making sure that your heel touches the pool bottom on each step. Land first on the ball of your foot and then let your heel roll down. You could hurt yourself if you stay on tiptoes. See Exercise 22.

Buttock kick jog
Jog with your heels kicking back toward the gluteal, or buttocks. Keep your body upright and your stomach muscles tight. See Exercise 5.

Jumping jacks
Do some jumping jacks in place, making sure that your toes and knees remain pointed in the same direction. Again, remember to get your heels down. See Exercise 32.

Moving jumping jacks
Move the jumping jacks forward and backward, covering the same distance as when you jogged. As you move forward, press your arms backward through the water. As you move backward, press your arms forward in the water. These arm motions help your body stay upright.

Cross-country ski

Take a position with your right foot forward and left foot back. Now switch, bouncing your left foot forward and right foot back. Bend your knees as you bounce, and bring your heels down. See Exercise 10.

Moving cross-country ski

Move the cross-country ski forward and backward through the water. At the same time, swing your arms forward and backward with elbows slightly bent.

Kicks

Do some kicks standing in place. As both feet come together during the bounce between each kick, make sure your heels touch the pool bottom and your knees are bent. Keep your shoulders back and your rib cage up while you're kicking. See Exercise 33.

Kneelifts

Switch to kneelifts, keeping the same speed, pressing your arms down and back through the water on each kneelift. See Exercise 35.

Moving kneelifts

Move the kneelifts forward and back through the water. Clap your hands behind your back as your knee comes up. As you back up, clap in front of your body instead of behind.

That's a good aerobic warm-up! By the end of 3 to 5 minutes of these exercises, you should be huffing and puffing a little, your heart should be beating faster, and you should feel warmer. You should feel like you've been exercising. If you feel as comfortable and relaxed as you did before you started, you need to pick up the pace, move the exercises a little farther, a little faster, and lift your knees a little higher.

Now you're ready for the main part of your workout. Chapter 4 includes a variety of aerobic exercises, chapter 5 takes you through the cool-down and poststretch, and chapter 6 takes you through muscle toning and strengthening exercises.

Remember, always include the thermal warm-up, prestretch, and aerobic warm-up before moving on to the exercises in chapter 4. Whether you decide to do water aerobics, water walking, or deep-water exercises for the aerobic portion, always protect yourself by warming up first.

WARM-UP SUMMARY

Do each exercise for 30 seconds. Hold each stretch for 5 to 10 seconds, and don't bounce.

THERMAL WARM-UP

Walk

Long-stride walking

Bent-knee walking

Tiptoe walking

Heel walking

Walk and roll

Side step

Side step with a dip

Low side step

Shoulder rolls

PRESTRETCH

Calf stretch

Hip flexor stretch

Hamstring stretch

Pectoral stretch

AEROBIC WARM-UP

Jog

High knee jog

Buttock kick jog

Jumping jacks

Moving jumping jacks

Cross-country ski

Moving cross-country ski

Kicks

Kneelifts

Moving kneelifts

CHAPTER 4

AEROBIC EXERCISES

Aerobic exercise serves several purposes. Exercising the heart and lungs enables you to function better in daily living. For example, exercising the heart and lungs gives you more energy to make it through the day or through busy times of the day.

Aerobic exercise builds a peripheral blood supply so that if some arteries become clogged, other arteries and veins are available. Exercising aerobically is extremely important.

Another reason it's important is the one that motivates most of us: It burns calories. Any one of these programs—water aerobics, water walking, deep-water exercises, circuit training, and interval training—will help you exercise aerobically and burn calories.

While you're doing any of the exercise programs described in this chapter, it's important to keep your legs moving. Don't stop to rest. Push yourself hard enough to huff and puff a little. It's also important that you don't become too fatigued, either in the muscles that you're using or in breathing. Remember, you're supposed to be smiling and having fun!

Many different exercise programs can be done in the water; I'll describe several of them. You can pick out a few that sound appealing to you. It's a good idea to vary the kind of exercises you do. Changing exercises every now and then provides better benefits. Just as if we eat a variety of foods, we're healthier if we do a variety of exercises. Varying your workout is called cross training.

Some people do one type of workout (water walking, for example) for 8 weeks, another type (water toning) for the next 8 weeks, and then a third type (circuit training) for 8 weeks before starting over. That's one way to cross train. Another is to alternate exercise types daily, doing water walking on Monday, water toning on Wednesday, and circuit training on Friday, repeating the sequence each week. Both methods work well, and make your workouts very effective.

Each of the following aerobic programs should follow the traditional format for an aerobics class, beginning with a thermal warm-up, prestretch, and aerobic warm-up; going on to the aerobic portion; and finishing with the cool-down, toning (optional), and poststretch.

WATER AEROBICS

Let's have some aerobic fun in the water! Do each exercise for 2 minutes unless otherwise noted. Remember that 20 minutes is the minimum time required to derive aerobic benefits.

*H*yperextension of the lower back means that your back is arched inward too much. This is very hard on the vertebrae in that part of the spine. Make a conscious effort to avoid performing any exercises in a hyperextended position.

Hopscotch
Do you remember hopscotch? You're going to begin with hopscotching to take you back to the fun and enjoyment of childhood. Begin by bouncing in place with your feet

shoulder-width apart. On every other bounce, lift one foot and land in the same imaginary square. The cadence goes like this: bounce, lift, bounce, lift. See Exercise 29.

1. Bounce with feet apart.
2. Bounce on the right foot, while lifting the left foot.
3. Bounce with feet apart.
4. Bounce on the left foot, while lifting the right foot.

Moving hopscotch

Hopscotch forward through the water. As you move forward, keep your stomach muscles tight and your hips directly under your shoulders to avoid hyperextending the lower back.

When we played this game as children, we'd turn around at the end and go back. In the water, to exercise all the muscles in a balanced way, you're going to back up rather than turn around. Lifting your foot behind you as you move backward through the water is challenging because the water pushes it forward. But go ahead and push your foot back as you lift it; this action works the back of your thighs. Remember to keep your feet shoulder-width apart.

1. Bounce forward with feet apart.
2. Bounce forward on the right foot, while lifting the left foot.
3. Bounce forward with feet apart.
4. Bounce forward on the left foot, while lifting the right foot.
5. Repeat several times, moving forward.
6. Repeat several times, moving backward.

Hop

In hopscotch, there are some single squares in a row, and you have to hop on the same foot through the row. Now you're going to practice hopping four times on one foot and then four times on the other. Go up on your toes when you push up. Bring your heel down to the pool bottom as you land. See Exercise 28.

1. Hop four times on the right foot.
2. Hop four times on the left foot.

Moving hop

Now move forward and backward just as with hopscotch. Keep your stomach muscles tight and your shoulders over your hips.

1. Hop forward four times on the right foot.
2. Hop forward four times on the left foot.
3. Hop backward four times on the right foot.
4. Hop backward four times on the left foot.

Vigorous moving hop

Increase the difficulty by using your arms more vigorously and by moving farther through the water on each hop. See Exercise 65.

1. Hop forward four times on the right foot, pushing the arms back forcefully on each hop so that you move forward as far as you can.
2. Hop forward four times on the left foot, pushing the arms back and moving forward as in Step 1.
3. Hop backward four times on the right foot, pushing the arms forward forcefully through the water, moving toward your starting point.
4. Hop backward four times on the left foot, pushing the arms forward and moving backward as in Step 3.

Jog

Jog in place for 1 minute, bringing your knees up high.

Side step

Walk sideways through the water, moving to the right for as many steps as space allows and then to the left for the same number of steps. As you step to the side, make sure your torso continues to face forward. Don't turn or look to the side. You should feel the inner thigh of the following leg working pretty vigorously. If you get tired, take smaller steps; if you want more exertion, take bigger steps. The following foot should come down right next to the lead foot. If you don't bring your feet together, you're not working the inner thigh as much as possible or burning as many calories as you could. See Exercise 53.

1. Step to the right with the right foot. Keep the right knee and toes facing forward.
2. Step the left foot over to the right foot.
3. Continue moving right.
4. Reverse direction, stepping off with the left foot.

Side step tilt

Continue side stepping, adding a movement that will help your midriff. I call this side step tilt. Remember, it's important to pull your feet together. It's also important that your shoulders tilt only to the side, not forward or backward at all. See Exercise 54.

1. Side step to the right, tilting the right shoulder down as you step.
2. Pull the left foot over to the right foot, straightening the torso.
3. Repeat several times.
4. Side step to the left, tilting the left shoulder down.
5. Pull the right foot over to the left foot, straightening the torso.
6. Repeat several times.

Leap

Now put a little bounce into your side step and leap sideways. As in the side step, go one way and then the other. When you leap to the right, your right foot always leads. When you leap to the left, your left foot always leads. Be sure your torso and legs face forward. See Exercise 36.

1. Lift the right leg to the side.
2. With a big jump, leap to the right and land both feet together.
3. Continue to the right until you run out of space.
4. Repeat the leaping move to the left.

Turn and leap

Instead of leaping sideways, you're going to turn and leap. When you leap to the right, face to the right. Always leap with the right leg leading. When you leap to the left, face to the left.

Always leap with the left leg leading. As you leap to the right or left, press both arms back forcefully through the water to move yourself forward. When you get good at this, you can pretend you're Mikhail Baryshnikov making high, bounding leaps. See Exercise 59.

1. Turn right.
2. Lift the right leg as high as possible.
3. Leap high and forward, landing on the right foot.
4. Step the left foot down.
5. Repeat several times.
6. Turn left.
7. Lift the left leg as high as possible.
8. Leap high and forward, landing on the left foot.
9. Step the right foot down.
10. Repeat several times.

Kick

Finish your water aerobics by standing in place and doing some chorus line kicks. Each time your foot comes down, be sure your heel touches the bottom of the pool. Lift your leg as high as you can. During each kick, keep your torso tall and stand upright. Leaning forward gives you poor posture and makes it harder to breathe. See Exercise 33.

1. Kick the right leg forward as high as possible.
2. Bounce with both feet together.
3. Kick the left leg forward as high as possible.
4. Bounce with both feet together.

One time through this workout provides the 20-minute aerobic minimum. You can repeat portions to make your workout as long as you want it. Remember to cool down and stretch.

WATER AEROBICS SUMMARY

Do each exercise for 2 minutes.

Hopscotch
Moving hopscotch

Hop

Moving hop

Vigorous moving hop

Jog (1 minute only)

Side step

Side step tilt

Leap

Turn and leap

Kick

WATER WALKING

Water walking is walking in waist-to-chest-deep water quickly enough to huff and puff. Change steps to ensure you use all the major muscles in the lower body. Walk forward, sideways, or backward. Point toes in or out. Bend legs or keep them straight. Walk on toes or heels. All these will vary the muscles used and help ensure a balanced workout. Use stroke, backstroke, figure eights, punching, and jogging movements to vary the muscles used in the arms, back, and chest. Modify intensity by changing arm movements or the direction of the walk.

To water walk with a low exertion level, all you need to do is slow down the step patterns. Don't move forward and backward very far. To water walk with a high exertion level, use lots of power on each step and move as far as you can through the water. Do each exercise for 2 minutes.

*L*ower leg, foot, and ankle injuries are not common in water exercise. If problems do occur, be sure to wear supportive shoes in the pool. You can also protect yourself from too much impact by moving into deeper water, adding a flotation belt or vest, or never bouncing off the pool bottom.

Regular walk

Walk in a normal stride. Keep your stomach muscles pulled in, ribs lifted, and chin back. Walk forward as far as you can. Then back up until you run out of space, and walk forward again. Walk normally, but with enough force to feel some exertion.

Walking the line

Keeping the same alignment, step one foot in front of the other so that you're walking a line. Lengthen your stride a little. Walk forward as far as you can and then back up, staying on the line. This is an excellent exercise for balance. See Exercise 68.

1. Step the right foot directly in front of the left.
2. Step the left foot directly in front of the right.
3. Repeat several times with a longer stride.
4. Reverse direction by stepping the right foot directly behind the left.
5. Step the left foot directly behind the right.
6. Repeat several times with a longer stride.

Crossing step

*I*f you've had hip replacement, check with your physician before doing the crossing step.

Stay on the line but crisscross your steps this time. At first you may need to shorten your stride to get the crossing motion in. As you get the feel for it and your hips begin to rotate side to side, you can lengthen your stride. Continue walking heel to toe, pushing yourself enough to huff and puff. When you finish the crossing steps moving forward, walk backward, crossing one foot behind the other. See Exercise 11.

1. Step the right foot in front of and across the left.
2. Step the left foot in front of and across the right.
3. Repeat several times with a longer stride.

4. Reverse direction by stepping the right foot behind and across the left foot.

5. Step the left foot behind and across the right foot.

6. Repeat several times with a longer stride.

High knee step

Go back to walking normally, but lift your knees up really high before you take a step. Use whatever arm motions you need to keep your balance. Bring the knees up as high as you can, and take as long a step as you can. See Exercise 24.

1. Lift the right knee as high as possible.

2. Take a giant step forward.

3. Lift the left knee as high as possible.

4. Take a giant step forward.

5. Repeat several times.

6. Reverse direction by lifting the right knee as high as possible.

7. Push the right leg down and behind you.

8. Lift the left knee as high as possible.

9. Push the left leg down and behind you.

10. Repeat several times.

High knee out

Vary the high knee step to work the inner and outer thigh. Continue walking with high knees, but point them to the side. Take a giant step forward. When you're backing up, lift the knee high to the outside and take a giant step backward. Straighten out your foot as it lands so it is not still pointing out. See Exercise 23.

1. Lift the right knee as high as possible to the right.

2. Take a giant step forward.

3. Lift the left knee as high as possible to the left.

4. Take a giant step forward.

5. Repeat several times.

6. Reverse direction by lifting the right knee as high as possible to the right.

7. Take a giant step backward.

8. Lift the left knee as high as possible.

9. Take a giant step backward.

10. Repeat several times.

Goose step

Change from a kneelift to a straight-leg lift. I call this the goose step. Lift your leg as high as you can, as if you're going to kick. Then step forward. This is not hard when you're moving forward. Wait until you try to back up! Continue to lift your leg as high as you can in front of you before you take the step back. The muscles in the back of your thigh and buttock will have to work very hard to pull your leg from a forward position into a step back. See Exercise 16.

1. Lift the right leg as straight and high as possible.

2. Take a giant step forward.

3. Lift the left leg as straight and high as possible.

4. Take a giant step forward.

5. Repeat several times moving forward.

6. Repeat several times moving backward.

Buttock kick

Step forward with your right foot. Pull the heel of the left foot up behind you as if you're trying to kick your buttock with your left heel. After the kick (or attempted kick!) swing the kicking leg forward, straighten it, and take a giant step forward. As your left foot steps forward, repeat the buttock kick with the right heel. After you've moved forward as far as you can or want, do the kick moving backward. First, pull the heel back and up, then straighten your leg backward to take a step back. This variation works the muscles in the front (quadricep) and back (hamstring) of the thigh. See Exercise 5.

1. Pointing the right knee at the pool bottom, lift the right heel behind the body toward the right buttock.

2. Straighten the right leg and take a giant step forward.

3. Point the left knee at the pool bottom, and lift the left heel behind the body toward the left buttock.

4. Straighten the left leg and take a giant step forward.

5. Repeat several times moving forward.

6. Repeat several times moving backward.

Side kick

Push your heel out to the side and up. You're doing a sidekick. Pull that foot in and take a giant step forward. Repeat with the other leg. Do the same kind of step when you back up. Push the leg up and out to the side and then pull it in and take a giant step backward. This exercise works the inner and outer thigh. See Exercise 52.

1. Push the right leg straight out to the side.

2. Pull the right leg in front of you and take a giant step forward.

3. Push the left leg straight out to the side.

4. Pull the left leg in front of you and take a giant step forward.

5. Repeat several times moving forward.

6. Repeat several times moving backward.

Power step

Continue with the side kick, but add a power dip. As you kick out to the side, straighten the other leg and go up on tiptoe. As you step forward, bend your knees and get low in the water. You should be as high as possible on the side kick and as low as possible on the step forward. See Exercise 44.

1. Go up on tiptoe with the left foot and push the right leg straight out to the side.

2. Pull your right leg in front of you and take a small step forward.

3. As the right foot steps forward, bend both knees until the shoulders are beneath the water surface.

4. Straighten the knees and push the left leg out to the side.

5. Pull the left leg in front of you and take a small step forward.

6. As the left foot steps forward, bend both knees until the shoulders are beneath the water surface.

7. Repeat several times moving forward.

8. Repeat several times moving backward.

Circle and step

*I*f you've had a hip replacement, check with your physician or therapist before doing this exercise.

Lift the right leg out to the side and back a little. Bring it around to the front in a half-circle motion and step in front of the left foot. Repeat with the left leg. Move slowly enough to get a nice big half circle. As you back up, you'll be doing the same thing, but you'll feel different muscles working. This works all the rotators in the hip and is excellent for hip mobility. See Exercise 9.

1. Lift the right leg to the back a little, and bring it out to the side and around to the front.

2. Step forward on the right foot.

3. Lift the left leg back a little, and bring it out to the side and around to the front.

4. Step forward on the left foot.

5. Repeat several times moving forward.

6. Repeat several times moving backward.

When you've finished these walking variations, you will have done a 20-minute aerobic workout. If you want a longer workout, repeat some of the variations. Remember to cool down and stretch.

WATER JOGGING

Some people like to bounce while they're moving through the water. If you prefer that kind of movement, you can change water walking to water jogging by bounding, bouncing, and leaping through the water in each of the walking exercises.

WATER WALKING AND WATER JOGGING SUMMARY

Do each of the following exercises for 2 minutes.

Regular walk

Walking the line

Crossing step

High knee step

High knee out

Goose step

Buttock kick

Side kick

Power step

Circle and step (This exercise should only be included in water walking programs. It is not intended for use in water jogging programs.)

DEEP-WATER WORKOUT

Deep-water workouts are so named because that's where the workout takes place—in the deep water, as in over your head.

Deep water is a very safe place to work out because there's absolutely no impact during the workout; your feet never touch bottom. Your muscles get excellent toning, and your heart and lungs an excellent aerobic workout because of the water's resistance.

To do this kind of workout, you'll need flotation equipment. With the equipment on, you should be suspended at about armpit depth.

There are different kinds of flotation equipment you can use. Flotation belts fasten around your waist. There's a wide variety of belts on the market; you should select one that's comfortable and stays in place. Flotation vests cover the torso. They are a little more expensive but seem to work very well. Flotation ankle cuffs go around your feet or ankles and hold you up just like the belt. Ankle cuffs are very comfortable but should not be used if you have balance problems. You need to be able to keep your feet under you when they're buoyant!

Do each exercise for 2 minutes.

*L*eaning forward for a long time stresses the lower back. Stay tall and maintain good body alignment. If you find yourself leaning forward, you're probably trying to move too quickly. Slow down and straighten up.

High knee jog

Begin by jogging in place with knees high. Bring each knee up as high as possible and push it down until your leg is completely straight. Use whatever pace works for you. If you want more exertion, bring the knees up a little higher and move a little faster. See Exercise 22.

1. Jog forward with the right foot.
2. While stepping on the right foot, pull the left knee up as high as possible.
3. Jog forward with the left foot.
4. While stepping on the left foot, pull the right knee up as high as possible.
5. Repeat several times.

Moving high knee jog

Continue high knee jogging. When you get to the end of the pool, jog backward rather than turning around. Backing up ensures a balanced workout and helps coordination and agility. In deep water, you may be tempted to lean forward as you move. Try to resist. Stay upright, with ribs lifted and shoulders over your hips.

1. Jog with knees high, moving forward several times.
2. Use breaststrokes, moving both arms at the same time.
3. Jog with knees high, moving backward several times.
4. When moving backward, one arm reaches back as the opposite knee comes up and pulls forward as the leg pushes down and back.

Crossing jog

*I*f you've had a hip replacement, check with your physician or therapist before doing this exercise.

Do high knee jogging, moving right and left, crossing your knee toward the opposite hip as you pull your knee up. Jogging with knees coming up and across works the hip rotators.

1. Cross the right foot over the left and "step" on it.
2. Jog the left foot to the left side of the right foot and "step" on it.
3. Repeat several times, moving left while facing forward.
4. Cross the left foot over the right and "step" on it.
5. Jog the right foot to the right side of the left foot.
6. Repeat several times, moving right while facing forward.

Bicycle
Bicycle in place while you rest your upper body. Pretend you're riding a bike, making a full circle with your feet on the pedals. See Exercise 3.

1. Pull the right knee up as high as possible.
2. Push the right heel forward and down.
3. As the right leg is pushing forward and down, pull the left knee up as high as possible.
4. Push the left heel forward and down.

Moving bicycle
Now move the bicycling action forward and backward. When moving forward, use overarm (crawl) strokes, but keep your

torso upright. As you move backward, use backstrokes. Your arms should windmill while your legs bicycle.

1. Pull the right knee up as high as possible, stretching the left arm forward.
2. Push the right heel forward and down, pulling the left arm back.
3. Pull the left knee up as high as possible, stretching the right arm forward.
4. Push the left heel forward and down, pulling the right arm back.
5. Repeat this several times, moving forward.
6. Pull the right knee up as high as possible, reaching back with the left arm.
7. Push the right heel down and back, pulling the left arm forward.
8. Pull the left knee up as high as possible, reaching back with the right arm.
9. Push the left knee down and back, pulling the right arm forward.

Cross-country ski

The cross-country ski is done in place. It feels different when your feet don't touch bottom! As one leg swings forward, the other one swings back. To keep your upper body stabilized, your arms need to swing opposite the legs. Your right leg and left arm should swing forward together. Keep your knees slightly bent. To protect the lower back, do two things: First, keep your stomach muscles tight and hips tucked. Second, keep your legs close to your body; don't swing them all the way forward and all the way back. Your legs should be doing the work but not swinging your upper body around in an uncontrolled way. See Exercise 10.

1. Begin with ankles together and the legs straight down from the hips.
2. Swing the right leg and left arm forward slightly.
3. At the same time, swing the left leg and right arm backward slightly.

4. Bring legs and arms to the beginning position.

5. Swing the left leg and right arm forward slightly.

6. At the same time, swing the right leg and left arm backward slightly.

7. Return legs and arms to the beginning position.

Moving cross-country ski

Now move forward and backward with the cross-country ski. It'll be a little bit more challenging, but still very enjoyable. The arm motion is the same, but you'll need to cup your hands to pull back powerfully for forward motion and forward powerfully for backward motion. Keep your body upright.

1. Begin with arms down, ankles together, and the legs together straight down from the hips.

2. Swing the right leg and left arm forward.

3. At the same time, swing the left leg and right arm backward.

4. Pull the right leg and left arm backward, cupping the left hand.

5. At the same time, swing the left leg and right arm forward.

6. Pull the left leg and right arm backward, cupping the right hand.

7. To back up, cup the hands in the opposite direction and push the arms forward.

Jumping jacks

This exercise looks like jumping jacks, but your feet don't touch down. Swing both legs to the side at the same time, then bring them together at the same time. This leg action makes your body bob up and down in the water. Be sure you're buoyant enough that your head doesn't go under! Your arms can swing in and out with your legs. Start easily, moving your legs a little out and in, without much power. When you have the hang of it, put some force into your moves. Push your legs out explosively and pull them back forcefully. This exercise works the inner and outer thigh. See Exercise 32.

1. Begin with ankles together and the feet straight down from the hips.

2. Swing the legs apart.

3. Squeeze the legs back together.

Buttock kick jog

Jog in place, but rather than bringing your knees up in front of you, keep them pointed toward the pool bottom. Keep your heels coming back and up behind you as though you're going to kick your buttock. This works the front and back of your thighs. See Exercise 5.

1. Pointing the right knee at the pool bottom, lift the right heel up toward the right buttock.

2. Straighten the right leg and lift the left heel up toward the left buttock.

3. Repeat several times.

Moving buttock kick jog

Move forward and backward with the buttock kick jog, using your arms for propulsion. As you do this exercise, you may notice your knees coming forward. To work the intended muscles, keep your knees pointed at the pool bottom, your heels kicking back, your ribs lifted, and your stomach muscles tight. The benefits of doing this exercise with correct technique are wonderful: First, you'll be working the muscles in the front and back of the thigh. Second, as your stomach muscles work to keep your torso upright, you'll get stomach toning with your aerobic workout!

1. Pointing the right knee at the pool bottom, lift the right heel up toward the right buttock.

2. At the same time, stretch the right arm forward.

3. Straighten the right leg. Simultaneously lift the left heel up toward the left buttock.

4. At the same time, pull the right arm forcefully through the water and stretch forward with the left arm.

5. Straighten the left leg. Simultaneously lift the right heel up toward the right buttock.

6. At the same time, pull the left arm forcefully through water.

To extend this workout beyond the 20-minute minimum, repeat any or all of the exercises.

DEEP-WATER WORKOUT SUMMARY

Do each of the following exercises for 2 minutes.

High knee jog

Moving high knee jog

Crossing jog

Bicycle

Moving bicycle

Cross-country ski

Moving cross-country ski

Jumping jacks

Buttock kick jog

Moving buttock kick jog

INTERVAL TRAINING

Interval training is a highly effective exercise method, but you need to be very well conditioned to use it. If you're interested in interval training, the water aerobics, water walking or jogging, or deep-water workouts can be modified for this purpose.

*I*nterval training is intended only for the very fit. Do not attempt it until you've been exercising without any problems for at least 8 to 12 weeks. Start slowly, with only 15 or 20 seconds of all-out effort. Work at moderate intensity for the rest of the segment, and then try all-out effort again. Do only 10 or 20 minutes of intervals the first time. If you have no problems the next day, you can begin to extend the duration of your workout.

To modify any of the workouts in this chapter for interval training, do the first 2-minute exercise at medium intensity. In the next 2-minute exercise, start with all-out effort for the first 30 seconds. Do the remaining 1-1/2 minutes of the exercise at low-to-moderate intensity. Do the first 30 seconds of the next exercise at all-out effort. Finish with 1-1/2 minutes at low-to-moderate intensity.

If you find that 30 seconds is too long for all-out effort, start with 20 seconds; finish the remainder of the 2 minutes at moderate intensity. Gradually increase the high-intensity portion of the exercise.

There are several ways to achieve all-out effort.

- Increase your range of motion by moving your limbs farther.

- Increase your force by putting more muscle power into each move.

- Increase your speed by moving faster. Be careful to maintain good posture and technique.

- Increase the height of your spring. Push off the bottom harder if you're doing water aerobics. Bend your knees, pushing up on each step during water walking. Push your body up and out of the water on each step in a deep-water workout.

- Increase your distance in each moving step.

INTERVAL TRAINING SUMMARY

Interval training can be used with water aerobics, water walking or water jogging, or deep-water workouts. Do the exercises in any of these programs in the order listed. Do the first 2-minute exercise at medium intensity. In the rest of the exercises, do the first 30 seconds with all-out effort; do the last 90 seconds at low-to-medium intensity.

The following summary uses the water aerobics program as an example.

Hopscotch: 2 minutes, medium intensity

Moving hopscotch: 30 seconds, all-out; 90 seconds, medium intensity

Hop: 30 seconds, all-out; 90 seconds, medium intensity

Moving hop: 30 seconds, all-out; 90 seconds, medium intensity

Jog: 30 seconds, all-out; 90 seconds, medium intensity

Side step: 30 seconds, all-out; 90 seconds, medium intensity

Side step tilt: 30 seconds, all-out; 90 seconds, medium intensity

Leap: 30 seconds, all-out; 90 seconds, medium intensity

Turn and leap: 30 seconds, all-out; 90 seconds, medium intensity

Kick: 30 seconds, all-out; 90 seconds, medium intensity

If you want to work out longer, repeat as much of the sequence as desired.

CIRCUIT TRAINING

Circuit training allows you to burn calories and tone muscles in the same workout. If you're interested in this kind of program, you'll combine the water aerobics in this chapter with the toning exercises in chapter 6. It's fun to add circuit training to your repertoire and use it for several weeks before switching workouts to cross train.

*A*ll movements should be slow and controlled, never fast and jerky. Remember to cool down and stretch before stopping.

After you've finished the warm-ups, do the first water aerobics exercise for 2 minutes. Next, move to the pool edge and do the first toning exercise at light intensity. Then, do the second water aerobics exercise for 2 minutes. (Be sure to use some exertion during the aerobic portion.) Go back to the pool edge and do the second toning exercise at light intensity. Continue to alternate aerobics and toning until you've done all the exercises in both programs.

A common error in circuit training is to move to the pool edge so slowly or to do the toning so easily that you lose aerobic benefits. Jog or move with a purposeful stride to the pool edge. Keep the intensity up. While toning, use as much muscle power as possible so you don't cool down. After toning, jog back to your position for aerobics. Make sure you continuously feel like you're getting a good workout.

CIRCUIT TRAINING SUMMARY

Hopscotch: 2 minutes

Upper arm toning: 8 to 10 repetitions

Moving hopscotch: 2 minutes

Chest and upper back toning: 8 to 10 repetitions

Hop: 2 minutes

Shoulders and sides of back toning: 8 to 10 repetitions

Moving hop: 2 minutes

Stomach, midriff, and back toning: 8 to 10 repetitions

Vigorous moving hop: 2 minutes

Front and back of thigh toning: 8 to 10 repetitions with each leg

Side step: 2 minutes

Outer and inner thigh toning: 8 to 10 repetitions with each leg

Side step tilt: 2 minutes

Front of hip and buttock toning: 8 to 10 repetitions with each leg

Leap: 2 minutes

Shin toning: 8 to 10 repetitions with each foot

Turn and leap: 2 minutes

Calf toning: 8 to 10 repetitions with each foot

Kick: 2 minutes

CHAPTER
5

COOL-DOWN AND POSTSTRETCH

The cool-down, muscle toning (or strengthening), and poststretch are the final parts of the workout. They're the parts I always look forward to! The cool-down and poststretch are required after every aerobic workout. Toning/strengthening is optional. If you feel like toning, you can; otherwise, you can skip it.

COOL-DOWN

*T*he cool-down is vital to your health. It's important that the lungs, heart, and muscles all cool down adequately. The cool-down can prevent muscle soreness, injuries, and heart stress.

After every workout, you should cool down for at least 5, and preferably 8 or 9, minutes. The cool-down brings your heart rate down and the systems in your body slowly back to normal. If you don't slow down gradually, you can create muscular, respiratory, and cardiac problems.

The cool-down is especially important in water exercise. While you're exercising, your blood is circulating rather quickly. Because the water pressurizes your body, your blood vessels could dilate and make you feel dizzy or lightheaded if you get out right after your aerobics. An adequate cool-down should prevent this.

During the cool-down, you should start to breathe more slowly and not as deeply as the lungs cool and gradually relax. You should be huffing and puffing less. Your heart rate should start to come down. This allows circulation to the muscles, heart, and brain to slow down. Your muscles should feel less tired.

The cool-down is my "thank you" to myself for exercising. It's when I congratulate myself and think of how much better I'll be during my next workout.

COOL-DOWN MISTAKES

There are some common mistakes made during cool-down.

- Taking a break, even for 30 seconds. Keep moving as you switch from high-intensity aerobics to the slow, low-intensity cool-down.

- Skipping the cool-down, going straight to poststretch. The heart and lungs are still working very hard. The muscles are still full of blood. It's very hard on your heart to get the blood moving again when it's pooled in the muscles. The muscles help the blood to flow, thereby helping the heart, if you keep moving slowly.

- Using short, small movements during the cool-down. It's important to use long, fluid, relaxed movements while cooling down. Let the muscles work all the way, not just in short patterns.

Now you know the purpose and importance of the cool-down. How do you do it? Here's a good routine. Do each exercise for 1 minute unless otherwise noted.

Power walk
Start by walking through the water. As you take each step, bend your knees, submerge your shoulders, and push up and

out of the water as you move to the next stride. This keeps the muscles in the legs working fairly hard but slows your heart and lungs because the pace and stride are relaxed. See Exercise 45.

1. Lift the right leg to the side.
2. Bring the right leg in front of you and take a small step forward.
3. Put the right foot down, bending the knees until the shoulders are under water.
4. Straighten the knees and lift the left leg to the side.
5. Bring the left leg in front of you and take a small step forward.
6. Put the left foot down, bending the knees until the shoulders are under water.
7. Repeat several times moving forward.
8. Repeat several times moving backward.
9. Continue for **2 minutes**.

Side step

Do some sideways walking (chapter 4). Walk sideways, going right and then left, as far as you can. See Exercise 53.

1. Step to the right with the right foot. Keep the right knee and toes facing forward.
2. Step the left foot over to the right foot.
3. Continue moving right. Reverse direction, moving left.
4. Continue for **2 minutes**.

Walk and roll

You'll recognize this exercise from the warm-up. The difference here is the length of your stride: Make these easy. Walk forward, rolling heel to toe. When you can't walk any farther, walk backward toe to heel. Make sure you go through the full roll on each step. This exercise focuses on some of the muscles in the feet and lower legs. See Exercise 67.

Duck walk

*I*f you've had hip replacement, check with your doctor before doing this exercise.

Walk with your toes pointed out, moving forward and backward. This will give you some extra hip rotation work before you quit for the day. You may look and feel like Charlie Chaplin, but I guarantee it's good for hip mobility. See Exercise 12.

1. Step forward with the right foot, toes pointed to the right.
2. Step forward with the left foot, toes pointed to the left.
3. Repeat several times, moving forward and backward.

Kneelifts

Do kneelifts in place, alternating your right and left knees. As you lower your leg, push with moderate force to get the leg all the way down and straight. Don't make this exercise too casual. See Exercise 35.

Long-stride walking

Long-stride walking is walking with as long a stride as possible forward and backward. Keeping your strides long stretches all the muscles in your legs. Leading with your heel as you're stepping forward stretches some of the muscles in the back of the lower leg. See Exercise 38.

Long-stride side step

The last cool-down exercise is sideways walking with long strides. Stretch your legs as far apart as possible and then bring them together. Move as far to the right as you can before going left. See Exercise 37.

TONING/STRENGTHENING

Your muscles should be relaxed and comfortable after the cool-down; your heart rate and your breathing pattern should be closer to normal. Now you have two choices. If you've done as much as you want, you can skip the toning and do the poststretch. If you feel like doing more, you can include some toning or strengthening exercises while your muscles are still warm enough to be challenged. It's a good time to include some muscle work if you're interested.

If you want to tone or strengthen, read "Toning with aerobics" in chapter 6 and do some of the exercises. Then do the poststretch in this chapter. It's very important to do the poststretch exercises at the end of every workout.

THE POSTSTRETCH

I think the poststretch is a bonus that just feels good, but there are physical reasons to include it. It promotes long-term flexibility: Poststretching helps you reach back to zip a zipper, reach up to the top shelf, or reach down to tie your shoes. The poststretch is also important because it may help to decrease muscle soreness from exercising. Finally, it finishes the cool-down, allowing the muscles to fully relax and stretch out and the heart and respiration rates to return to a resting level.

As you can tell, I feel the poststretch is not only fun, but very important. All well-qualified fitness instructors will take you through a 3-to-5-minute poststretch at the end of every workout.

STRETCHING PRECAUTIONS

Poststretching should be done with attention to the same precautions required in prestretching.

- Hold the stretches without bouncing or moving.
- Hold the stretches for at least 10 to 20 seconds each. Part way through, take a deep breath, relax all your muscles, and stretch a little farther. You can "breathe, relax, and stretch farther" two or three times if you hold the stretch long enough.
- Keep your muscles warm. If you start to cool down too much, and the muscles feel tight instead of limber, go back to some of the cool-down exercises for 2 or 3 minutes.

Intersperse cool-down movements with stretches until you're through all the poststretch exercises.

For the poststretch, use all of the prestretch exercises in chapter 3. To refresh your memory, these were

- calf stretch (page 38),
- hip flexor stretch (page 39),
- hamstring stretch (page 39), and
- pectoral stretch (page 40).

The following stretches should also be used. They should be held for 10 to 20 seconds.

Quadricep stretch

Face the pool edge and grab your ankle behind your buttock. Point your knee down and hold. This is similar to the position used to stretch the hip flexor, but there the knee is swung back a little, and the hip is pushed forward. In this stretch, the knee points down and the hip joint is relaxed. If grabbing your ankle behind you is uncomfortable, stand with both hands on the pool edge, lift your heel up as high as you can behind you, and point your knee straight down. See Exercise 46.

Gluteal stretch

Stand sideways to the pool edge, holding on with one hand. Hook the other hand under your knee. Pull your leg up and your knee toward your chest. Straighten your torso, pull your knee in a little tighter, and hold. Repeat with the other leg. See Exercise 15.

Midriff stretch

This stretches the oblique muscles, which are in the midriff. Stand with your torso completely upright without leaning forward or to the side. With your hands on your hips, twist from the middle of your torso to one side and hold. Keep your knees and toes pointed forward. You can bend your knees a little to keep them in the correct position. Now twist to the other side and hold. See Exercise 40.

Head and neck stretches

These next stretches are for the head and neck. It is very important to do these stretches after water exercise because the head is the only part of the body not buoyed by the water.

A word of caution regarding these stretches. Rolling your head around in circles, even at slow speed, could be dangerous. Eliminate full neck circles from your workout. They are very hard on the small vertebrae in the neck. For this reason, the various functions of the neck are separated and addressed by stretching the muscles one at a time rather than in a circling motion.

1. Tilt your head so that your right ear goes down toward your right shoulder. Relax, let it go as far as possible, and hold. Straighten up, relax in the straight up position, then let your left ear go down toward your left shoulder and hold. See Exercise 19.

2. With chin back and head upright, turn your head to look over your right shoulder and hold. Face forward, relax in that position, then turn to look over your left shoulder, and hold.

3. Rest your chin as far down as you can on your chest. Relax and let your head hang forward. Let the muscles in the back of the neck stretch out. Hold, then bring your chin up and relax. See Exercise 20.

Upper body stretches

Now for some upper body stretches. If you start to get chilled during these stretches, you can walk through the water while you're doing them.

1. Interlace your fingers and stretch both arms forward in front of your face. Turn your palms out and stretch as far forward as you can. You should feel an easy stretch in the upper back. Hold. See Exercise 62.

2. Pull your right arm across your chest at shoulder level, using your left hand. Press your right elbow toward your chest.

You should feel a stretch in the back of the right shoulder and upper back. Hold, then repeat with your left arm. See Exercise 64.

3. Interlace your fingers, palms up, and press both arms up as high as you can. Lift from the midriff and make your middle as small as possible. Hold. See Exercise 61.

4. Lower your arms behind and above your head and grasp your elbows with the opposite hands. Hold. See Exercise 63.

Joint exercises
These three exercises, while not stretches, also improve flexibility. They are smooth, continuous motions of short duration.

1. The first exercise is for your shoulder joint. Roll your shoulders forward, then up, then back, and around. Continue for 10 to 20 seconds. To reverse, roll your shoulders backward, then up, around to the front, and back again for 10 to 20 seconds. See Exercise 48.

2. The second exercise is for your wrist joint. Rotate your wrist, making a big circle with your fingertips. After 10 to 20 seconds, go the other way. See Exercise 31.

3. The third exercise is for the ankle joint and some of the bones in the foot. Put some weight on the ball of one foot, keeping the heel up. Make circles with your ankle in one direction for 10 to 20 seconds, then reverse. Repeat with the other foot. See Exercise 30.

At this point you should be cooled down, stretched out, and relaxed. You may exit the pool safely. Be sure you use the ladder or stairs and watch your footing.

Now that you've finished your workout, notice how you're feeling. Do you feel tired or exhilarated? Do you have more energy, or are you drained? If you feel exhausted, you may have worked too hard. The next time that you exercise, go a little easier. You should be able to leave your exercise session feeling exhilarated and with renewed energy.

Relaxation

If you have a warm-water pool (86 degrees Fahrenheit or warmer) and you're interested in doing some relaxation exercises, this is an excellent time. One technique for relaxation is to tense and relax each part of the body. Starting at the lower part of the body, tense the lower leg as hard as possible, squeezing the muscles as much as you can with as much force as possible. Hold that contraction for 10 to 20 seconds. Next, completely relax these muscles and stay relaxed for 20 seconds. Move up to the thighs, contracting all the muscles in the upper legs as hard as you can. Hold for 20 seconds, then relax. Move up to the buttocks, stomach muscles, chest and back muscles, upper arm, lower arm, and neck. Contract, hold, and relax each group. You can do the full progression or specific muscle groups as you choose. If you don't have a warm-water pool, relaxation exercises probably won't be comfortable.

Flexibility

Some people are only interested in a flexibility program, not in aerobics. For a flexibility program, you need to be sure all the muscles are warm. Go through a full thermal warm-up as described in chapter 3. It's not necessary to do the prestretches because you'll be moving straight into the flexibility stretches. As soon as you're warmed up, start the stretches in this chapter. Hold them for at least 60 seconds.

If you're doing a flexibility program, you will probably have a pool that's 88 to 92 degrees. Becoming chilled is unlikely, but if you start to feel cold, do the thermal warm-up exercises again before moving on to more stretches.

All of the stretches in a poststretch can be used in a flexibility program. However, in the flexibility program, stretches are held for a longer period of time, usually about 60 seconds in total. There are several ways to accomplish this.

Option one
Go through the poststretch exercises, holding each for 60 seconds.

Option two

Go through the poststretch exercise sequence once, holding each stretch for 20 seconds. Repeat the sequence two more times.

Option three

Go through the poststretch exercises. Stretch the calves first, 20 seconds on the right leg, 20 seconds on the left leg, and repeat twice. Stretch the right hip flexor muscle for 20 seconds, the left for 20 seconds, and repeat twice. Continue through all the stretches in this way.

COOL-DOWN AND STRETCH SUMMARY

Do the following exercises for 1 minute.

Power walk

Side step

Walk and roll

Duck walk

Kneelifts

Long-stride walking

Long-stride side step

(Toning/strengthening, if desired.) Hold each of these stretches for 10 to 20 seconds.

Calf stretch

Hip flexor stretch

Hamstring stretch

Pectoral stretch

Quadricep stretch

Gluteal stretch

Midriff stretch (twist)

Head and neck stretches

Upper body stretches

Joint exercises

CHAPTER 6

TONING AND STRENGTHENING EXERCISES

On some days you may just want to tone or strengthen muscles with no aerobics. On other days you may want to add toning or strengthening to your aerobic workout. This chapter guides you through either choice.

As I explained in chapter 1, muscle tone (also called muscle endurance) determines your ability to repeat resistance activities many times. Increasing muscle tone gives your muscles the ability to endure. When you push your grandchild on a swing, you'll be able to push longer. When you help out on the assembly line making food packages for the homeless, you'll be able to keep going longer and with greater ease. Chapter 4 described several aerobic programs. Those programs are aerobic because they cause you to take in more oxygen. They condition heart and lungs. They cause you to burn more calories.

This program is anaerobic, much like the flexibility program in chapter 5. But that doesn't mean you don't burn calories. While an aerobic program improves the function of your heart and lungs by working them, the anaerobic program improves the function of your muscles by increasing their tone and strength.

Muscle strength is being able to pick up or move a heavy object one time. Building muscle strength gives your muscles more power. When it's time to vacuum behind the sofa, you'll be able to move it more easily. When you swing your golf club or lift your grandchild, you'll be able to put more power into the movement. Whichever you decide to work on, you'll improve both. You'll also notice a more toned look to your body no matter which you use.

As you can tell from these examples, both muscle tone and strength are important. It used to be thought that the ability to build muscle tone and strength was lost with age. As the following study shows, that's not true. No matter how old or out of shape we are, our bodies will improve when we work our muscles. Muscles do tend to lose strength with age, but the decrease can be slowed or even reversed with regular resistive exercise.

In the study, six women and four men began strengthening exercises at the Hebrew Rehabilitation Center for the Aged in Boston. The 10 frail participants were between 90 and 96 years of age and had the following health profiles.

- Each had four or five chronic diseases (arthritis, diabetes, etc.).
- All needed medications four or five times a day.
- Seven had osteoarthritis.
- Six had coronary artery disease.
- Six had suffered stress fractures (cracked bones) from osteoporosis.
- Four had high blood pressure.
- Seven regularly used a cane or other walking device to get around.
- All took a long time to stand from sitting in a straight chair.
- Eight had a history of falls related to muscle weakness.

These individuals seemed unlikely to benefit from exercise, or even to be able to exercise!

But after participants exercised within their abilities for 8 weeks, the researchers from several area universities and hospitals concluded that "a weight-training program is capable of inducing dramatic increases in muscle strength in frail men and women. . . ." Translated, that means these 10 individuals improved so much that even the researchers were shocked!

The participants gained an average 174% in strength after just 8 weeks. That means that if a participant had been able to lift only a half cup of coffee without shaking at the beginning of the study, they'd be able to lift almost two full cups without shaking after 8 weeks. If they started out needing a walker to help their legs support half of their body weight, they ended with legs that could do the job by themselves! Their muscle size increased and that means their strength improved. Best of all, their mobility improved. They were able to get out of chairs faster with more confidence. They were able to get around better.

If we're going to be alive, we might as well be kicking! We might as well be able to get around and do things. Working on muscle tone and strength will help us achieve that.

How to Use the Program for Muscle Toning or Strengthening

The basic program has different results, depending on the workout level and the number of repetitions you choose. You'll use the same exercises for toning or strengthening; the only differences will be whether or not you work with equipment and how much force you use. When you work without equipment with light force for more than eight moves (repetitions), you'll be improving muscle tone. When you work with equipment such as webbed gloves, barbells, or ankle cuffs with heavy force for fewer than 15 repetitions, you'll be improving muscle strength.

Each exercise in this chapter can be done at light, moderate, or advanced levels.

- Light—8 to 10 repetitions using easy movements
- Moderate—15 to 20 repetitions without equipment; 8 repetitions with equipment
- Advanced—Same number of repetitions as moderate level but with forceful movements

TONING

To use this program to tone, go through the thermal warm-up and prestretch. Do the exercises in this chapter at the light-to-moderate level. After you've done these exercises once, repeat them at least once, preferably twice. Ideally you'll be doing three sets of each exercise. Then do all of the poststretch exercises (chapter 5).

TONING WITH AEROBICS

If you're adding a toning segment to your aerobics program, do it between the cool-down and the poststretch. Go through each one of these exercises at the light-to-moderate level one time. You may do more if that's your preference. Then do the poststretch exercises (chapter 5).

TONING GUIDELINES

Here are some guidelines to follow when doing toning exercises.

• Do not bounce during the exercises; you'll get better muscle tone.

• Isolate the working muscles. This means the muscles used in the exercise should be the only ones moving. If the rest of your body "wags," you're doing the exercise too quickly or moving the limb too far. You'll know that your speed and range are right if you can keep the muscle group you're working isolated.

• Stop and start each movement. A common mistake people make in toning is to use a fluid motion. When you're toning, you need to think about where the limb is going and stop it when you reach that point. Then rest and start the next movement. If you get to the end of one movement and come back without stopping, the muscle fibers won't use as much energy. The toning won't be as good, and the caloric consumption won't be as great. Be sure to stop at the end of each movement.

STRENGTHENING

To use this program for strengthening, use equipment with each exercise in this chapter. Do the thermal warm-up and prestretch first. Then do the exercises in this chapter at the advanced level, all the way through, once. Repeat the series two more times for a total of three sets. Finally, do the poststretch exercises (chapter 5). It is very important to do all the stretches.

THE TONING AND STRENGTHENING PROGRAM

Thermal warm-up

Begin by walking in the water for about 5 minutes and practicing good posture as you did in chapter 3. Be sure you're comfortable with the water, the pool bottom, and the temperatures of the water and your body before you go on to the prestretch.

Prestretch

Use the prestretches in chapter 3. Gradually stretch out some muscles, then walk some more before stretching other muscles. Once you've finished the prestretch, you're ready to tone or strengthen.

Upper arm

Working the biceps (in front) and triceps (in back) of the upper arm improves your ability to lift things (grocery bags, babies, bowling balls, luggage) close to your body, to hit a tennis ball, and to push things (sofa or lawn mower). See Exercise 60.

1. Begin with the arms at sides, palms facing up.
2. Bend the elbows (but keep them in at the waist) and lift the hands toward the shoulders.
3. With the hands still up at the shoulders, turn the palms out and press the hands straight down to where they started.
4. Turn the palms forward.

For advanced level—Moderate-level repetitions but pull up as hard as you can, rest while you're turning your palms, then press down as hard as you can.

Chest and upper back

Chest and upper back muscles help you hug other people, stand up taller and straighter, and keep your shoulders and neck free from aches and pains. See Exercise 8.

1. Begin with the arms extended sideways in the water, palms facing forward.
2. Press the arms toward each other until they meet in front of the chest.
3. Pull the arms away from each other, returning to the beginning position. Squeeze the shoulder blades together as you do this.

For advanced level—Moderate-level repetitions but press your arms together as strongly as possible, rest, then pull them apart with all your strength.

Shoulders and sides

Shoulder and side muscles help pull the garage door down, push the garage door up, reach out to pull the car door shut, and lower or raise window blinds. See Exercise 50.

1. Begin with arms at the sides, palms facing the thighs. Bend the knees a little to get the shoulders in the water.
2. Lift the arms out sideways to the top of the water. The palms face down.
3. Bring the arms straight down, back to the beginning position.

For advanced level—Same as moderate-level repetitions but

*H*anging from your shoulders on a pool edge or from kickboards, using your arms overhead too much, or moving your arms in and out of the water too frequently can all lead to shoulder problems. Nerves and tendons in the joint can become pinched. If your shoulders start to bother you, stay away from all hanging exercises, and keep your arms in the water during the entire workout.

lift your arms up and out as strongly as possible, rest, then push them down with all your strength.

Stomach, midriff, and back
Strengthening the stomach, midriff, and back muscles allows you to twist more safely, as when you reach for the seat belt in the car; lean forward more safely, as when you pick something up; stand taller; and look thinner. You will be able to sit up from lying down more easily. See Exercise 57.

1. Stand with the back to the pool edge and the elbows in the gutter.
2. Rest your weight on the arms and tuck the knees in toward the chest.
3. Press the small of the back against the pool wall while swinging the hips slightly forward.
4. Lower the hips and relax the back.

For advanced level—Do this exercise 15 to 20 times. Rest your shoulders. Do a second and third set of 15 to 20 repetitions each.

Front and back of thigh
The front and back of the thigh are the muscles that help you walk and bend. They also help you to stand from a sitting position, to straighten your legs when pulling pants on, and to kick a ball when you're playing kickball with the kids. See Exercise 14.

1. Stand sideways to the pool edge.
2. Hold on to the pool edge with one hand and lift the opposite knee.
3. Straighten the knee.
4. Bend the knee, keeping it pointed forward, and pull the heel back toward the hip.
5. Repeat according to work-out level.
6. Repeat with the other leg.

For advanced level—Moderate-level repetitions but straighten your leg as forcefully as possible, rest, then bend your knee with all your strength.

Outer and inner thigh

The outer and inner thigh muscles help you move sideways as through a narrow spot. They help you to cross your legs and to pick up your feet to put on socks. See Exercise 41.

1. Stand sideways to the pool edge and hold on with one hand.
2. Lift the outside leg to the side, about 12 to 15 inches. Keep the toes pointed forward.
3. Pull the leg back down through the water.
4. Repeat according to workout level.
5. Repeat with the other leg.

For advanced level—Moderate-level repetitions but lift your leg to the side as forcefully as possible, rest, and pull it back with all your strength.

Hip and buttock

*I*t is important to keep your knee joint stationary as you lift and lower the leg. It's also important that your leg be relatively straight. Lowering your leg could stress your lower back if your technique is poor. Before lowering your leg, pull your stomach in. Pulling your stomach in protects the lower back.

These muscles (the front of the hip and the buttock) help you with normal, everyday movements such as walking, going up stairs, getting up from a table at a restaurant, and getting out of bed. See Exercise 25.

1. Stand sideways to the pool edge and hold on with one hand.
2. Put all your weight on the foot closest to the pool wall.
3. Lift the outside leg forward as far as possible without leaning forward.
4. Lower the leg.

5. Repeat according to workout level.

6. Repeat with the other leg.

For advanced level—Moderate-level repetitions but lift your leg as forcefully as possible, rest, then lower it with all your strength.

Shins

The muscles in the shins help you walk, lean forward, and lift your foot when you're tying your shoes. These muscles help to stabilize and strengthen the ankle joint. See Exercise 47.

1. Stand sideways to the pool edge and hold on with one hand.

2. Put one foot slightly forward of the other.

3. Keep the heel of the forward foot on the pool bottom and lift the toes as high as possible.

4. Lower the toes.

5. Repeat according to workout level.

6. Repeat with the other foot.

For advanced level—Moderate-level repetitions but lift your toes as forcefully as possible, rest, then press your toes down with all your strength.

Calf

The muscles in the calf help you walk, go up on tiptoe, and bounce. These muscles help to stabilize and strengthen the ankle joint. See Exercise 6.

1. Stand facing the pool edge and hold on with both hands.

2. Position the feet close to the pool wall.

3. Go up on tiptoe on both feet, keeping the torso upright. Be sure the legs rather than the arms are supporting your weight. Arms are used to maintain balance.

4. Lower the heels to the pool bottom.

For advanced level—Moderate-level repetitions but go up on your toes as forcefully as possible, rest, then press your heels down with all your strength.

TONING AND STRENGTHENING SUMMARY

Do each of the following exercises at a light, moderate, or advanced level.

Upper arm

Chest and upper back

Shoulders and sides

Stomach, midriff, and back

Front and back of thigh

Outer and inner thigh

Hip and buttock

Shins

Calf

CHAPTER 7

POSTREHABILITATION EXERCISES

Special exercises to help some physical conditions can be added to the other programs in this book. I'll review a few of those conditions and the exercises recommended for them.

WHAT IS POSTREHABILITATION?

Postrehabilitation (postrehab) refers to people who have been through physical therapy and rehabilitation and are ready for an at-home program. If you're fortunate, you may find a postrehab program at your community pool. This program is offered by aquatic instructors who have also trained as aquatic therapy technicians. It is important that you get the approval of your physician and/or physical therapist before taking part in an organized program. It is even more important that you get approval before trying the workout in this chapter on your own.

One of the benefits of postrehab water exercise is improved balance in the water. Whether you're standing, sitting, or moving, you'll have better balance.

Postrehab water exercise also allows for a greater variety of movements than you would be able to do on land.

Postrehab water exercise can

- enhance independence,
- increase strength,
- increase flexibility,
- increase circulation, and
- prevent muscles from weakening.

Postrehab water exercise is especially beneficial because it can increase the speed of recovery. Whether you've had a broken bone, a hip replacement or stroke, or simply have tight muscles, you can recover faster in the water.

WHO CAN BENEFIT FROM POSTREHAB WATER EXERCISE?

This program is for anyone with one or more of the following conditions and who has already been through a physical therapy program. If you have weakness, pain, decreased range of motion, limited mobility, swelling, or a loss of balance, this program is ideal for you. It can also benefit someone with arthritis, multiple sclerosis, tendinitis, total knee replacement, total hip replacement, and back injuries.

WHO SHOULD NOT USE THIS PROGRAM?

This program is not intended for anyone who has not been through a physical therapy program or who has open wounds, bowel or bladder incontinence, or infection. Anyone who has had a tracheostomy should probably not participate in water programs since water in the trachea can cause drowning. Anyone who has a temperature of over 100 degrees is advised not to use this program.

HOW IS IT DONE?

Begin your postrehab program by going through the thermal warm-up and stretching exercises in chapter 3. Since this is not an aerobic program, you do not need to include the aerobic warm-up. After stretching you can begin the therapeutic exercises that are comfortable for you, starting with the upper body and moving down.

*T*hese exercises are not intended to be done vigorously. They are intended to work your muscles easily to loosen and lubricate your joints. They are also intended to move your joints as far as they can comfortably go. If you feel a pain or catch in a movement, make the movement smaller.

Shoulder shrugs
See Exercise 49. If your shoulders ache, bend your knees or kneel so that your shoulders are below water.

1. Lift the shoulders toward the ears.
2. Relax them.
3. Repeat this exercise 8 to 12 times.

Wrist circles
See Exercise 31.

1. Put the hands and wrists in the water.
2. Rotate the wrist, making a big circle with the fingertips.
3. Stop and rotate in the opposite direction.
4. Repeat 8 times.
5. Repeat with the other hand.

Finger touches
Open your hand and touch your thumb to the tip of each finger. Exercise both hands at the same time. See Exercise 13.

1. Touch the index finger with the thumb.
2. Open the hand and touch the middle finger with the thumb.
3. Open the hand and touch the ring finger with the thumb.
4. Open your hand and touch the little finger with the thumb.
5. Repeat 8 times.

Your spine can twist so you can look behind you and to the side. Your spine can bend to the side so you can tilt sideways and forward so you can bend forward. Do each of those moves separately. Never combine them. For example, if you're bending forward, don't twist at the same time.

Midriff
See Exercise 40.

1. Stand with hands on hips, feet shoulder-width apart, and knees relaxed.
2. Twist from the waist (not the knees) toward the right.
3. Return to center position.
4. Twist from the waist to the left.
5. Return to center position.
6. Repeat 8 to 12 times.

Side bends
See Exercise 51.

1. Stand with hands on hips, feet shoulder-width apart, and toes pointed slightly out.
2. Lean from the waist toward the right side.
3. Straighten up and pause.
4. Lean from the waist toward the left side.
5. Straighten up.
6. Repeat 8 to 12 times.

Stomach
See Exercise 56.

1. Walk forward in a big circle.
2. Stop and do a pelvic tilt every 8 steps.
3. When you are comfortable with the pelvic tilt and the walking, try to do the pelvic tilt on the eighth step without stopping.

4. Repeat until you've done 8 to 12 pelvic tilts.

Note: The pelvic tilt is explained in chapter 3 in the hip flexor stretch. If you find it difficult, try the "sponge squeeze." Imagine a water-filled sponge in your stomach. Using your stomach muscles to squeeze the water out tilts the pelvis forward.

Upper and lower leg

This is a good mobility exercise. See Exercise 35.

1. Stand in place.
2. Lift the knee up as high as possible.
3. Lower it and lift the other knee.
4. Repeat 16 to 20 times.

Hips

Keep this nice and easy. Your leg should be the only thing moving. This is also a good mobility exercise. See Exercise 27.

1. Stand sideways to the pool edge and hold on with one hand.
2. Circle the leg from the hip 8 times in one direction.
3. Rest.
4. Circle 8 times in the opposite direction.
5. Repeat with the other leg.

Knee circles

See Exercise 34.

1. Keeping the torso upright, stand with your back to the pool edge.
2. Lift the knee up to the chest.
3. Hold the leg up with hands under the thigh if necessary.
4. Circle the lower leg from the knee 8 times in one direction.
5. Rest.
6. Circle 8 times in the opposite direction.
7. Repeat with the other leg.

Ankle circles
See Exercise 1.

1. Keeping your torso upright, stand with your back to the pool edge.
2. Lift one knee toward the chest. Hold it there with both hands under the thigh.
3. Circle the ankle 8 times in one direction.
4. Rest.
5. Circle it 8 times in the opposite direction.
6. Repeat with the other leg.

Ankle flex
See Exercise 2.

1. Stand sideways to the pool edge.
2. Point the toe of one foot like a ballerina until it's pointed as far as it can and you feel stretch on the top of the foot.
3. Pull the toe up toward your face as far as you can until you feel stretch in the back of the ankle.
4. Repeat 8 to 12 times.
5. Repeat with the other foot.

WHAT'S NEXT?

You're not done yet! These exercises are just the beginning. If you feel good, you can do the toning exercises in chapter 6 at the light level. Then do all the poststretches in chapter 5 as listed.

Now you're done! You should feel great, and it's safe for you to exit the water.

PART

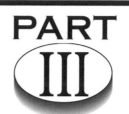

III

CREATING YOUR PROGRAM

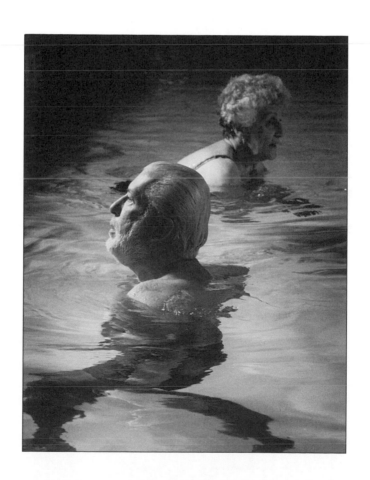

CHAPTER 8

IDENTIFYING YOUR NEEDS

No two people are exactly alike. We all have different physical capabilities, and we all want different things from our exercise programs. It's important that you tailor your program to your individual needs. The first step is to identify what you want your program to achieve.

CHOOSING THE RIGHT PROGRAM

If you don't create your own program, and if more than one class is offered in your area, making the right choice can take some thought. Here are some guidelines to help you choose a program that's right for you and that's safe and effective.

Goals—The underlying goal of exercise is functionality. This means, at the minimum, that exercise will help you function better in daily life. Whether your goal is to be able to get on your hands and knees to scrub the kitchen floor or to become fit enough to run a marathon, increased functionality is the purpose. Simply exercising will help you achieve better functionality. Specific exercises and exercise programs help to achieve other goals such as losing weight, toning muscles, and improving balance and coordination. Choose the class that works what you want to work.

Convenience—Is the class offered in a facility that's easy to get to? Is it offered at a time that fits your schedule? Can you use the facility during nonclass times to exercise on your own?

Cost—The right class should fit your financial situation. Classes in North America cost from $.50 to $25 per class. The average fee is $5.

Safety—All the programs in this book follow a safe format. An aerobics class should begin with a thermal warm-up and prestretch for 5 to 10 minutes (longer if the water is cold), then move to the aerobic warm-up. The aerobics exercise portion should last at least 20 minutes nonstop, and your legs (not just your arms) should be moving continuously. The cool-down should last about 5 minutes, followed by toning (if it's included), and the class should finish with a flexibility segment.

Intensity should be monitored. Heart rates or perceived exertion should be checked during the class to be sure aerobic conditioning is taking place and calories are being burned.

The pool should be clean, safe, and comfortable. The deck should have a nonskid surface, and the locker room should be well maintained.

There should be a lifeguard on duty and an emergency action plan posted.

Variety—Muscle balance cannot be achieved using only kicks and kneelifts. Exercises should move your limbs and make your body go forward and backward and side to side. Arm movements should be included with leg exercises.

Instructor—The instructor should have Aquatic Exercise Association or comparable certification. This means the person is knowledgeable about general exercise (basic anatomy, kinesiology, and exercise physiology); the laws of physics and how they apply to water exercise; pool, water, and air specifications; program guidelines; leadership; emergency training, basic water rescue, and injury prevention; water exercise equipment use and precautions; nutrition and weight loss; and legal issues.

The instructor should be aware of your current health status. Do you have a special situation that might require program modifications? If you do, the instructor may be able to guide you in adapting the class program to your needs. If the instructor can't help, use the modifications described in chapter 9. If you can't find a program that meets your health status needs, you may need to create your own following the ideas found in this book.

The instructor should be professional, should dress and speak appropriately, and should put the interests of the class first. The instructor should be willing to work with your doctor or therapist in selecting and adapting exercises for you. Class should begin and end on time. It should be motivating, effective, safe, enjoyable, and educational.

If your program meets these criteria, you can be assured of a safe, effective workout.

WHAT'S BEST?

There are different types of programs for different fitness needs. As I mentioned, your muscles may be strong, but you may become short of breath. Or your breathing may be fine, but your muscles may feel exhausted after a short time. Use the following descriptions to choose the type of program that matches your fitness needs and goals.

WATER AEROBICS

If you're interested in burning calories, losing weight, and being able to last longer when carrying the groceries in, a water aerobics class is the type to look for. This class includes moving your body through the water and moving your legs and arms enough to make you huff and puff.

Participating in a class like this usually results in weight loss and a general feeling of improved health.

Although not geared toward toning, a water aerobics class benefits tone because you work against the water's resistance.

WATER WALKING AND WATER JOGGING

If you're just starting to exercise, consider a water walking program. Water walking achieves aerobic benefits by using simple step variations. If you enjoy bouncing, it's easy to modify water walking to water jogging. Since both programs are aerobic, they help you burn calories and lose weight.

Neither is geared toward toning, but exercising against the water's resistance improves muscle tone.

DEEP-WATER WORKOUT

If you've had recent surgery on your legs or feet, or you're recovering from a lower extremity injury, it may be best to exercise in water that's deep enough to keep your feet from touching bottom. A flotation belt, vest, or ankle cuffs will keep your head above water. The wonderful thing about deep water is that your feet, ankles, knees, hips, and back never absorb any impact. This type of workout is extremely gentle to the body.

INTERVAL TRAINING

If you feel that you are already quite fit and want a challenging workout, look for an interval training program, sometimes called intervals. This type of program alternates long periods (2 minutes) of low-to-moderate intensity aerobics with short periods (30 seconds) of extremely high-intensity aerobics. This kind of class burns calories! You will also gain muscle tone from working against the water's resistance.

CIRCUIT TRAINING

If you want to combine muscle toning and aerobics, look for a circuit training class. Circuit training interposes toning exercises between 2- to 3-minute aerobic segments. By the end of each session, you will have toned most of your major muscle groups while burning the same number of calories as in an aerobics workout. If you can't find a circuit training class, you can create your own by jogging for 3 minutes, toning for 1 minute, and repeating several times.

TONING

If you're mostly interested in having firm, sleek muscles, look for a toning class.

This program usually involves various leg exercises at the pool edge and arm and abdominal exercises farther out in the water.

In a toning class you'll be moving parts rather than your whole body. You won't be getting an aerobic workout or burning a lot of calories.

ABDOMINALS

If you want to flatten your stomach, you may be able to find a class specifically for these muscles. This type of class involves toning at the pool edge, some standing stomach muscle exercises, and some that use flotation equipment.

This class too has no aerobics portion and is not intended to burn calories.

Table 8.1 summarizes typical class characteristics for each of these programs.

WHAT IF THERE'S NOTHING OUT THERE?

If you are unable to find a program that meets your needs, you can create your own using the information in this book. To maintain your current fitness level, use any of the programs in this book. To improve your fitness level, use any of the programs and periodically increase one aspect of your workout.

FITT

Whether you want to maintain or improve your fitness, you'll need to understand the FITT principle. FITT stands for frequency, intensity, time, and type.

I'll describe each element of FITT, how to use it to maintain your current fitness level, and what to do if you want to improve it.

Frequency is the first element. Frequency means how often you exercise each week. The minimum weekly frequency required to maintain or improve fitness is three. That means you should begin by exercising at least three times a week on nonconsecutive days. The day or days between each exercise session allows your body to rest.

Intensity is the second element. Intensity is tested either by heart rate or by rate of perceived exertion. The minimum

Table 8.1

Typical Class Characteristics

Class Type	Aerobic Benefits	Muscle Toning	Duration (minutes)	Class Size	Cost per Session	Facility Type
Water aerobics	Y	Some	40-60	20-40	$4-10	Shallow water
Water walking	Y	Some	40-60	15-25	$3-10	Shallow water, comfortable bottom
Water jogging	Y	Some	40-50	15-30	$4-10	Shallow or deep water
Deep-water workout	Y	Some	40-60	15-25	$3-10	Deep water
Interval training	Y	Some	40-50	20-30	$4-10	Shallow or deep water
Circuit training	Y	Y	45-60	10-20	$5-15	Shallow water
Toning	N	Y	20-40	10-15	$2-5	Shallow warm water
Abdominals	N	Y	15-30	10-15	$2-4	Shallow warm water

requirement for aerobic improvements is either "somewhat hard" on the perceived exertion chart (p. 27) or 105 to 145 beats per minute. Work up to that level and then stay there in order to maintain your current fitness level.

Time is the third element and refers to the duration of each exercise session. Twenty minutes is the minimum duration for effective exercise. If you have been very inactive, you may need to work up to 20 minutes.

Type is the fourth and final element. It's important that the types of exercise you do use the legs and be continuous and rhythmical. The aerobics programs in chapter 4 all meet these criteria.

Now you can apply the FITT principle to the exercise program you create: No matter which program you choose, exercise at least three times a week, work out at the minimum intensity level as measured by heart rate or rate of perceived exertion, and include at least 15 minutes of nonstop movement.

If you can't start at these levels, don't panic! It's okay to work up to them gradually. By following any of the programs in chapter 4 to meet these minimums, you'll improve your current fitness level if you've been sedentary in the past. If you've been active, meeting these minimums will help you maintain your current fitness level.

MAKING PROGRESS

After following your program for 8 weeks, you may realize you feel so good that you want to continue improving. To improve, use one of the FITT elements to increase the challenge of your workout. For example, if it's convenient, increase your exercise frequency to four times a week. Or increase the intensity of each workout, making a greater effort each time you exercise. If you're happy with the frequency and intensity of your workout, increase the duration by 5 minutes each time you exercise. Or, finally, change the type of exercise you're doing. If you've been water walking for 8 weeks, switch to a deep-water workout. Remember to change only one element at a time, as shown in Table 8.2.

Over the course of 5 months, you will have increased the challenge of your program in four different ways. If you're happy with your exercise program and fitness level, continue your program as it is. If, however, you want to improve your

Table 8.2

		Using FITT to Change Your Program		
Week	Frequency (per week)	Intensity	Time (minutes)	Type
1-8	3	Somewhat hard	15	Water walking
9-12	4	"	"	"
13-16	"	Heavy	"	"
17-20	"	"	20	"
21-?	"	"	"	Water aerobics

fitness level, continue changing your workout according to the FITT principle.

You can also use the FITT principle in a toning or strengthening program. Increase the challenge of your workout by increasing the number of workouts each week (frequency); the number of repetitions, muscle force, or equipment used (intensity); the length of the workout (time); or the kind of exercises you do (type).

EXERCISE GUIDELINES

You've determined your needs and located a class or created your own program. Do you know everything you need to? Not quite. The following guidelines will protect you from exercise problems.

- Work to the point of tension, not pain. Your muscles and body should feel the effort, but the effort should not be painful.

- The 2-hour pain rule applies. If, 2 hours after exercising, you have more pain than before you exercised, you probably attempted to do too much during the session. Do less during your next workout.

- If you experience pain during your workout, stop exercising.

- Work toward good muscle balance. Most muscles are

paired and one of the pair is usually stronger than the other. You should strengthen and stretch both muscles in the pair. The exercise programs in this book are designed to do that.

- Your knees and elbows should always be slightly bent. Avoid locking these joints; it puts too much stress on them.

- Don't clench your facial muscles, jaws, arms, hands, or anything else. Clenching reduces blood flow to the muscles and can increase blood pressure. Keep your body relaxed and move easily.

- Avoid jerky movements. Protect your muscles and joints by exercising in a smooth, controlled manner.

- Even though you're breathing faster and deeper, breathe naturally and comfortably. Do not hold your breath during any of the exercises. Holding your breath prevents your muscles from getting the oxygen they need. It can increase blood pressure and put undue stress on the heart.

- Use good shoes. Water exercise shoes cushion some of the impact and make the workout easier on your joints. They protect you from slipping by gripping the pool bottom, and keep you from rubbing the bottom of your feet raw.

- Choose a good water depth. Begin in shallow water (hip-to-waist depth). As you become accustomed to exercising in water, you may want to move out deeper to give yourself more buoyancy and less impact stress. The correct water depth lessens the likelihood of injury. Midriff-to-armpit depth seems to be ideal for most people.

- Find a good water temperature. You may need warmer than average water to keep your body core temperature up if you are doing a very basic workout. You'll probably find 84-to-90-degree Fahrenheit water ideal for that level of exercise. Water temperature in the mid-80-degree range seems to be ideal for people who can exercise in vigorous aerobics programs.

- If you're a beginner, stay away from water exercise equipment. Weights, resistance equipment, and buoyant equipment should not be used until you've exercised successfully with no problems for 8 to 12 weeks. The exception is flotation equipment to keep you buoyant in deep water.

PROPER BODY ALIGNMENT FOR EXERCISING

Maintaining good posture (body alignment) is important. The human body is designed for movement; when properly aligned, it is unlikely to break down with use. Correct posture balances the weight of your body which, in turn, avoids overworking any muscles.

A properly aligned body looks like this: From the front, if an imaginary line were drawn down the center, your body would be equal on both sides. The center of the hip joint, the center of the knee, and the center of the ankle should all be in a straight line. Of course, you will move out of this position for some exercises, but it is important to return to it between exercises.

From the side, the ear should be centered over the shoulders, and the shoulders over the hips. This is extremely important for safety. Leaning forward or letting your head lean forward puts undue stress on the back muscles.

Here are some techniques for maintaining good alignment:

1. Let your shoulders drop away from your ears. Shoulders move up from stress or if the water temperature is too cool. Relax your shoulders and upper back muscles.

2. Make a conscious effort to keep your rib cage up. This not only brings you into good alignment, but also allows your lungs to work more effectively.

3. Imagine the string of a helium balloon coming out of the top of your head, lifting the weight of your head for you.

4. Allow your arms to move naturally if no specific arm movements are given for an exercise.

5. Move easily and naturally through the water. Only challenge yourself if you can maintain good alignment. Leaning forward is a sign that you're trying to move too far or too fast.

6. Stand tall. Imagine how you look from the front and side. Visualizing yourself standing tall will help you stay aligned.

CHAPTER 9

WITH YOUR CONCERNS IN MIND

Some of you may have medical concerns, needs, or conditions that require modifications in your exercise program. In this chapter, I address some of the most common situations. I can't emphasize enough the importance of regular physical check-ups, clearing your exercise program with your physician and therapist, and calling your physician or therapist with any minor problems you encounter from exercise. Sometimes we think our problems are normal (and most of them are!). But there are other times when a normal problem combined with a special situation can alert your doctor or therapist to the need for closer consideration of your condition.

ARTHRITIS

In the past, individuals with arthritis have been cautioned to stay away from any type of exercise that might irritate their condition. However, pain and stiffness in the joints can be decreased through low-to-moderate intensity exercise. Exercise will actually make you feel better! The lubrication of the joints that occurs during the thermal warm-up (chapter 3) is good for them and can make exercise pleasurable rather than painful.

There are two major types of arthritis: osteoarthritis and rheumatoid arthritis. Although they are separate conditions, the exercise modifications are the same.

Go through the thermal warm-up twice before moving on to the prestretch. Your joints and muscles will appreciate the longer warm-up period.

Be sure to take time to enjoy both stretching segments of the workout and feel free to stretch for longer periods of time than suggested. Stay away from hard stretches that may put too much pressure on your joints. By keeping the stretches comfortable, you'll protect the joints.

The exercise programs in chapters 5 and 6 concentrate on using large muscles and the major joints (elbows, knees, hips). You may want to include some exercises for the smaller joints (wrists, fingers, ankles) in chapter 7. Just make sure you're moving the joint in every direction possible for you.

Bouncing should be eliminated from any program that you do. This means that water aerobics is probably not the program for you. Instead, try the water walking program or the deep-water program.

Ideal water temperature for people with arthritis is 88 to 92 degrees Fahrenheit. You may be able to exercise comfortably in cooler water if you wear a full unitard, wet suit, or a wind surf suit.

To protect your joints, don't use equipment during the first 8 to 12 weeks of any exercise program.

Any exercises that hurt while you're doing them should be stopped immediately. If you are having an inflammatory episode, a flareup, or you have hot joints, you may want to check with your doctor before exercising that day. If you do exercise, the affected areas should be submerged in the water, since water naturally reduces swelling.

You'll know that you exercised too much if 2 hours after your workout, your body hurts more than usual. If this happens, take at least 1 day off and then do a shorter, less intense workout the next time.

FIBROMYALGIA

Fibromyalgia is a condition in which muscles ache nonstop. People with this condition experience muscle pain all over, are tired most of the time, are afraid to do anything physical (including exercise), and sleep poorly.

No cure exists for fibromyalgia, only techniques to relieve the painful symptoms. Recommendations usually include taking warm baths; applying heat; massage; following a regular sleep schedule; sleeping 8 hours a night; avoiding alcohol, caffeine, and tobacco before bedtime; taking midday naps if possible; using relaxation techniques; and, surprisingly, exercise.

Regular workouts help people with fibromyalgia become more fit, more flexible, have better blood flow to the painful muscles, and achieve better posture. The most important things to remember when working out are to maintain good posture and to keep your workout easy.

Good posture in the workout is vital. This helps align the muscles and allows you to feel comfortable standing tall. Fibromyalgia can be made worse by exhausting the muscles. Avoid muscle fatigue by keeping your workout intensity low and taking rest breaks if necessary.

A low-intensity water walking or deep-water program would be ideal and could markedly improve your symptoms. At first you may only be able to do a 5-minute warm-up. Gradually add 1 to 3 minutes a week. The intensity should not increase. Try to build up to 20 to 30 minutes of exercise three times a week.

Do the thermal warm-up twice and then do the prestretch gently. The prestretch makes exercise more comfortable and prevents injuries. The water walking workout should be perfect for you.

Finish your workout by doing the cool-down twice before the final flexibility portion.

OSTEOPOROSIS

Osteoporosis, which means porous bones, is a condition in which the bones become progressively more fragile and likely to cause pain or break. As you age, your bones gradually lose some of the minerals that make them strong. Smoking, crash diets, and extreme thinness also speed bone mineral loss. The best example of osteoporosis is a dowagers hump, a rounding of the spine just below the neck. The effects of osteoporosis are also seen in the number of hips broken during falls.

Two things, regular exercise and a diet rich in calcium, can retard bone mineral loss. Moderate regular exercise will retard, and sometimes reverse, osteoporosis. It used to be thought that the exercise had to be weight bearing and impact producing (walking, running, aerobic dance) to have a beneficial effect on bone density. Now we know that stress on the tendons, ligaments, and periosteum (the place in the bone where new bone cells are made) is what triggers an increase in bone density.

Bones that are not used weaken gradually. Bones that are subjected to responsible exercise become stronger. Forcefully pushing and pulling limbs through the resistance of water puts the right kind of stress on the bones.

If you have osteoporosis, water exercise can help. You can follow the water walking and deep-water programs without modification. Water aerobics involves a little more bouncing. If you want to use water aerobics but have a sore neck, back, or hips afterwards, you'll need to do it with less impact. Slide, rather than bounce, your feet through the movements.

Do the toning part of your workout at a moderate level in order to trigger cell creation. If possible, do the toning twice.

If you are in pain from osteoporosis, move to deeper water (armpit-to-shoulder depth) to lighten the load.

SHOULDER PROBLEMS

If you're experiencing shoulder problems, shoulder pain, or rotator cuff problems, you should exercise in water that's deep enough to keep your shoulders submerged. This alleviates some of the pain and impingement in the joint during exercise.

Do the thermal warm-up twice. The rest of the exercise program can be done as listed, but be sure to avoid any strength work with the upper body. Keep your arms in the water and never use any weights.

During the toning portion of the program, do not hang by your elbows from the pool edge. Skip the exercise (stomach, midriff, and back) that requires this position.

Move your arms easily and slowly. Keep shoulder joint movements short enough to avoid pain.

Knee and Hip Problems

A water environment is the perfect place for people with knee and hip problems. Here are some modifications that will make it even better.

Make sure that all of your movements are smooth, slow, and controlled. Avoid jerky movements involving the knees and hips.

Deep-water exercise is the ideal program for people with hip and knee problems. Water walking is a good alternative. The decreased bouncing will alleviate some knee and hip pain and most of the stress on the knees and hips. If you have had hip replacement surgery, don't do any exercises that cross one foot over the other without your physician's approval.

For both knees and hips, avoid any twisting exercises with the feet planted.

The toning exercises for inner and outer thigh, front of hip and buttocks, and front and back of the thigh should all be done carefully. These exercises should be done a second time to help strengthen and stabilize the knees and hips.

Lower Back Pain

Since the causes of back pain are so varied, it's impossible to give specific exercise modifications. These comments are very general.

- Stop any exercise that causes pain immediately.
- Eliminate fast twisting from your exercises.
- Use cushioned shoes to absorb impact during exercise.
- Use abdominal toning exercises (chapter 6) extensively. Intersperse them throughout your workout. Strengthening the abdominals protects the back and decreases lower back pain.
- Hold the hamstring muscle and hip flexor muscle stretches a little longer. Do them two or three times pre- and poststretch.

- Eliminate bouncing (water aerobics) from your program. The water walking and deep-water workouts would be excellent.
- Keep your arms in the water. Using your arms overhead can cause instability in the back.
- Exercise in water as deep as possible. The more buoyant you are, the less body weight your back will have to support.

OBESITY

If you are obese, your exercise session should last fairly long (30 minutes), and the intensity should be very low. Work up to 30 minutes gradually if you need to.

Exercise at least three times a week. After 8 weeks, you may increase the frequency to four times a week. Be sure that you have no aches or pains before increasing the frequency.

You need to keep impact on joints and connective tissue as light as possible. Use the water walking or deep-water program rather than water aerobics. Wear cushioned shoes for the water walking program to protect yourself from the small amount of impact involved.

Be cautious of overheating. If water and air temperatures are high, keep your intensity very low. If your breathing becomes labored, slow down and rest between exercises.

Use the thermal warm-up, prestretch, and aerobic warm-up as described in chapter 3. The aerobic portion should be followed as explained in chapter 4, but do each exercise an extra 15 to 30 seconds. Extend the cool-down at least one and a half or two times; give your body temperature time to decrease. The poststretch doesn't need modification.

DIABETES

Activity of any kind is very important for anyone with either Type I or Type II diabetes. Exercising improves insulin sensitivity, plasma and lipid profiles, and cardiovascular function.

If you deal actively with your diabetes, you should monitor your glucose level before and after a workout. Most doctors suggest that diabetics eat fruit or a couple of pieces of bread before exercise and then a meal or another snack after exercise. Check with your doctor to see if this is true for you.

It's very important to keep fluids in your body. Drink before, during, and after your exercise session. Juice diluted 1:1 with water is a good source of fluid and the carbohydrates that you'll need.

It's common for people with diabetes to suffer from a loss of sensation in the lower extremities. This means you might not be able to feel problems in your feet and legs. Because of this, you should never exercise barefoot; be sure to wear shoes during every workout.

As a diabetic, you should know your signs of hypoglycemia. If an attack occurs during exercise, most doctors suggest that you stop exercising, take carbohydrates (fruit, fruit juice, bread), wait 15 minutes, and then consider returning to exercise. Check with your doctor to see if you should follow these suggestions.

CORONARY ARTERY DISEASE

This topic includes angioplasty, coronary bypass, angina, atherosclerosis, ischemic heart disease, valve disease, cardiomyopathy, heart attacks, and all the other heart-related diseases. It's impossible to give specific modifications for so broad a range of conditions, but there are some general recommendations you should follow.

- Clear your exercise program with your doctor.

- Dizziness, chest pain, pressure, or angina all indicate a problem with the exercise session. Stop exercising and contact your doctor.

- Increase the amount of time spent on the warm-up. Do the thermal warm-up and prestretch as listed, but do the aerobic warm-up twice before moving into the aerobic exercise.

- Exercise with only moderate intensity during the aerobic portion. You should always feel comfortable during exercise.

- Water aerobics, water walking, or deep-water exercise can work well for you.

- Do not use the interval training program.
- Exercise at least three times a week. Gradually work up to four or five times a week if your physician approves.
- Keep your exercise session easy.
- Keep your session short. Skip some of the exercises so that your workout lasts only 20 to 30 minutes all together.

HYPERTENSION

Water exercise is extremely beneficial for hypertension. Regular exercise helps regulate blood pressure.

The thermal warm-up and prestretch should be done as indicated in chapter 3, and the aerobic warm-up twice. The best aerobic program choice is slow water walking. While it is important to exercise, it is also important to compensate for your high blood pressure while exercising. Keep your exercise intensity low. After the aerobic portion, do the cool-down exercises twice to be sure your body is returning to normal.

Do the toning portion with very light effort. Using a lot of force can increase blood pressure. Do the poststretch portion of the workout and then get out of the pool very gradually. You should feel no dizziness and no lightheadedness as you get out of the pool. If you do feel dizzy, stay in the water and walk slowly for a little while. Now you should be able to get out of the water without feeling lightheaded.

It is very important not to hold your breath during any exercise movement. It is also important not to use any exercise equipment. When your muscles contract from holding your breath, using force or equipment, or toning, the blood vessels constrict (get smaller) and blood pressure increases. Avoid forceful, tense, or explosive exercise movements.

STROKE

People who have had a stroke are often able to exercise in the water even when they are unable to exercise on land. If your leg muscles are weak, they may improve through a simple water walking program.

Water walking helps any leg muscles that have been affected. It helps to retrain you to walk on land; it reeducates your muscles and strengthens them. If you have trouble supporting your weight in the water, use a buoyant vest.

If portions of your upper body were affected by the stroke, it's important to get those areas submerged. Don't expect big movements and don't expect quick improvements. It takes time, but you will eventually improve.

If one of your limbs is nonfunctional, help it to move by using your other arm or your arms to move it. By being moved as it normally would, it may be able to regain some function.

Use the water walking program and concentrate on equalizing your strides (making each step the same length) even if you move slowly. Concentrate on keeping your torso upright and on standing tall.

You should wear water exercise shoes during water exercise to protect your feet in case you drag one of them.

ASTHMA AND OTHER BREATHING DISORDERS

People with breathing disorders usually find that water exercise is excellent for them. The warm, humid air in the pool environment makes exercise and breathing much easier.

It is important to increase the length of your warm-up. After finishing the thermal warm-up, repeat the second half. Do the aerobic warm-up exercises all the way through twice before going on to the aerobic portion of your workout. Interval training works well for people with breathing disorders.

Repeat the cool-down exercises until you've spent at least 10 minutes bringing your body back to normal. Take deep breaths during the cool-down, in through your nose and out through your mouth. Nasal breathing helps keep moisture in the air flow to the lungs.

You should avoid eating food for at least 2 hours before exercising. Sometimes food combined with exercise can trigger an asthma attack.

Most people who take medication for their breathing disorders should take it before exercising. Symptoms usually appear in the first half hour (and usually within the first 10 minutes) of exercising. Keep your bronchodilator or whatever medication you use at the pool edge in case you need it.

Most pool workouts will be ideal for you. However, if you do start to have symptoms, stop exercising immediately.

GASTROINTESTINAL PROBLEMS

People with gastrointestinal (GI) conditions should be able to exercise comfortably. When you exercise and breath deeply, several things happen to your GI tract. First of all, GI activity slows down. Because the body is so busy accommodating the exercising muscles, it can't get the usual amount of blood, enzymes, and hormones to the GI tract. This is good, because you certainly don't want to have GI disturbances during exercise!

There are several things you can do to avoid GI problems during exercise. The first one is to wait at least 2 hours after a meal before exercising. On the days you exercise, choose foods that are high in carbohydrates (such as bread) instead of fat or protein. If you're really hungry, but it's only 1 hour before exercise, choosing a liquid meal might help.

Drink plenty of fluids during exercise. It's important to drink water or low-sugar sports drinks rather than highly concentrated liquids like juices just before and during exercise.

Take plenty of time to warm up. If you're using one of the programs in this book, do the aerobic warm-up twice. Keep your exercise intensity level very low until you see how things work for you. When you decide to increase the intensity level, do so very gradually.

Moderate exercise can actually help GI tract problems. Keeping your exercise at low-to-moderate intensity should speed the passage of food through your stomach. Moderate exercise can also relax your mind, which helps the GI tract. The GI tract seems to work best when the mind is free from worry.

MEDICATIONS AND WATER EXERCISE

If you take medications regularly, ask your doctor if exercising will change the timing of your doses. Also ask if your medication will affect your exercise in any way.

Some common medications affect exercise heart rates or resting heart rates. I've made a list of those medications and their effects on heart rates (Table 9.1). Use this information and the information in chapter 2 about workout intensity to monitor your heart rate. If Table 9.1 shows that the medication you're taking lowers the working heart rate, you should not expect to achieve the numbers found on the heart rate chart (Table 2.5). If you push yourself to achieve those numbers, you could be harming yourself. The information about medications is very generalized and may not reflect your current situation. Always check with your doctor.

Table 9.1

Some Possible Effects of Different Medications on the Heart Rate Response

Medication	Effect on heart rate response
Beta blockers	decreased
Alcohol	no effect or increased
Digitalis	decreased or increased
Antihistamines	no effect or increased
Tranquilizers	no effect or decreased
Diet pills	no effect or increased
Cold medication	no effect or increased
Caffeine	no effect or increased
Nictoine	no effect or increased
Diuretics	no effect
Antihypertensives	no effect or decreased or increased
Calcium-channel blockers	no effect or decreased or increased
Antidepressants	no effect

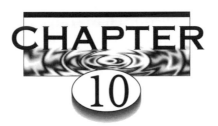

CHAPTER 10

TRACKING YOUR PROGRESS

Now that you have some complete exercise programs to follow, it's important that you track your progress. One of the reasons people stop exercising is that they don't notice the benefits. In order to stay motivated, you should track your progress so you can see exactly what benefits you have achieved.

SETTING AND ACHIEVING GOALS

Begin by setting one or two goals. These goals can be general or specific, short term or long term. A short-term general goal could be to have two people tell you you're looking better. A long-term general goal could be to have the energy to enjoy your grandchild during the day and still rest well at night by the end of 6 months of water exercise.

You may have more specific goals. A short-term specific goal could be to lose 5 pounds before a class reunion. A long-term specific goal could be improved blood pressure in 6 months. Another long-term specific goal could be to lower your resting heart rate to 72 beats per minute.

After you've set your goals, write them down on a progress chart. I've included a filled-in chart (Table 10.1) as an example. Make copies of the blank chart and write your goals at the top. Fill in your progress every week or two. Be sure to mark the date at the top of the columns (see Table 10.1). The chart covers 6 months for a good reason: Changes don't happen overnight. Give yourself time for the benefits to show up and also for some possible, and very human, backsliding.

Keep your chart visible and use it. Seeing your progress will help to keep you exercising regularly.

WATER EXERCISE LOGS

Another way to stay motivated to exercise is to keep an exercise log. Having a plan will help you stay on it and committed. Put as many details into your exercise log as you can. List who you exercised with, the time you went, how long you exercised, which exercises you especially enjoyed, and which ones you don't particularly like. List any problems you may have encountered during an exercise session. Definitely keep a record of any soreness that you have afterwards. The sample log (Table 10.2) will help you chart this information.

EVALUATE

After you've been exercising for a month or so, it's time to evaluate the program you're participating in. Reread chapter 8 and review the needs you had for an exercise program. If your program is meeting your needs, continue it. If your progress chart shows you're making progress, stay with your program. If, however, the program is not meeting your needs and the progress chart doesn't show much progress, you may need to make some changes. Keep an open mind about exercising. Don't assume that if you haven't made progress, exercise isn't for you; you may just need a different approach.

Maybe it's time to increase the challenge of your workout using the FITT principle. On the other hand, maybe your program is too challenging and you need to cut it back using the FITT principle. If your program is too challenging, you won't be enthusiastic about it and it could lead to injury. You

Table 10.1

Sample Goals Chart

GOAL 1: Feel better, happier or healthier.
GOAL 2: Lose 5 pounds.
GOAL 3: Improve blood pressure reading.
GOAL 4: Have more energy for grandchildren.
GOAL 5: Reduce resting heart rate to 72 BPM.

GOAL	1/15	1/30	2/15	2/28	3/15	3/30	4/15	4/30	5/15	5/30	6/15	6/30
1.	Feeling tired	YES! Feel better	Hooray! Feeling healthier									
2.		1 lb.	2 lbs. total	Still at 2 lbs.	4 lbs. Yipee	Still at 4 but almost there	Hooray! 5 lbs.	Write new goal to maintain				
3.	Dr. appt.	Next Doctor appointment in 5 months — May 16th								Dr. appt.	Blood pressure down!	
4.		Kids come June 1st for four days									Hooray! I did it. I love them so much.	
5.	RHR is 80 BPM		RHR is 78 BPM		RHR is 76 BPM							Hooray! 72 BPM

Table 10.1 *(continued)*

Goals Chart

GOAL 1:

GOAL 2:

GOAL 3:

GOAL 4:

GOAL 5:

GOAL											
1.											
2.											
3.											
4.											
5.											

A blank chart for you to copy and use.

Table 10.2

Weekly Exercise Log

Activity	Week 1			Week 2			Week 3			Week 4		
(Minutes)	M	W	F	M	W	F	M	W	F	M	W	F
Water walk	20'	15'	20'	15'	15'	20'	20'	15'	20'			
Aqua aerobics												
Toning	5'	5'		5'	20'		5'	10'				
Flexibility	5'	5'		5'	5'		3'	5'	3'	3'	3'	3'
Circuits	3'	3'	3'	3'	3'	3'				20'	20'	20'

Daily Exercise Log

Activity	Monday	Wednesday	Thursday	Saturday
Begin	9:00 No motivation	9:00 Too pooped for aerobics. Try toning today.	9:00 Ready to go!	9:00 Anxious to go. Not as strong today.
Thermal	9:15 Water cool at first.	9:15 Did twice to get going!	9:15 Strong & purposeful moves through this.	9:15 Good start. I always can get through this part.

Table 10.2 *(continued)*

Activity	Monday	Wednesday	Thursday	Saturday
Prestretch	9:20 Shoulder tight. Otherwise just right.	9:25 Oh yes!	9:20 Pushed each stretch to the limit.	9:20 Shoulder tight. No pain.
Cardio	9:22 Sluggish start. Got going by the end.		9:22 This was perfect. I was perfect.	9:22 I kept it easy today.
Aerobics	9:28 Walk program was fun!		9:28 1/2 aqua aerobics & 1/2 water walk. Loved it!	9:28 Water walk. Started easy, became an animal. I am awesome!
Cool-down	9:48 How relaxing!		9:48 Could have kept going. Cool-down felt good.	9:48 This was great.
Toning/strength	9:53 Was going to skip today. Did first half.	9:28 Did all twice. Had so much fun, did a third time.	Skipped today.	9:53 Second half of toning from Monday.
Flex	10:00 Limber today.	10:00 Tired muscles enjoyed stretch.	9:53 Listened to music. My body stretched perfectly.	10:00 Chilled so I kept them @ ten seconds— worked well.
After	10:05 I feel refreshed. More energy than an hour ago.	10:05 I feel strong. Glad I tried this.	10:00 "Crinky" shoulders looked "uncrinky" today.	10:03 From so-so to go-go day.

may feel frustrated, irritable, exhausted, and have trouble sleeping if you're working too hard. Remember that the water will always work with you, no matter what it is that you need. Try different aerobic or anaerobic programs. Try exercising at different times of the day. Try a new facility. Don't give up. The benefits of exercise are too valuable.

Go!

Water can help you achieve wonderful success with your health and fitness goals. It's kind, it's refreshing, it's rejuvenating, and it's fun. It will wake you up when you're tired and relax you when you're stressed. Whether you want a gentle workout or a challenging, forceful workout, water will accommodate you.

I hope I've convinced you to start, and continue, water exercise. Remember, those who do not find time for exercise, sooner or later, will have to find time for illness. Find the time to be healthy and happy—now!

PART
IV

EXERCISES
ILLUSTRATED

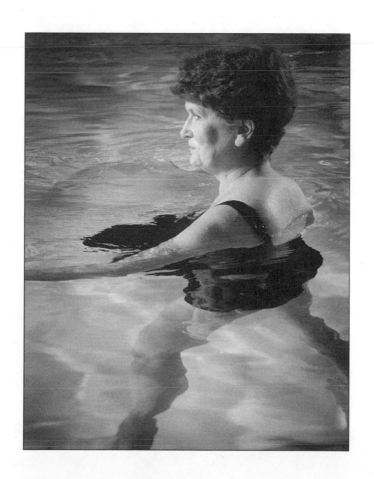

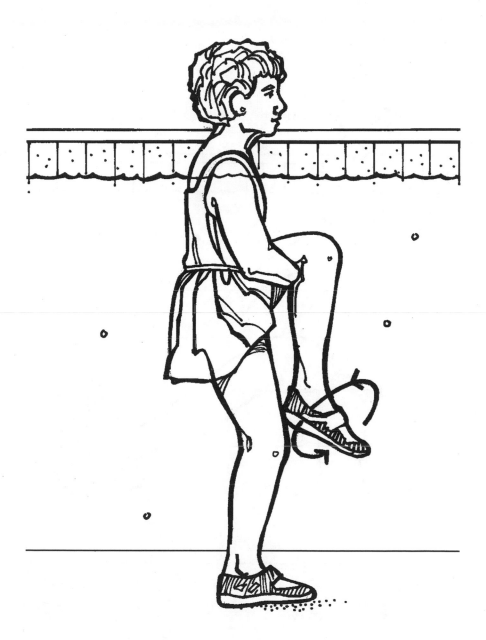

1.   ANKLE CIRCLES

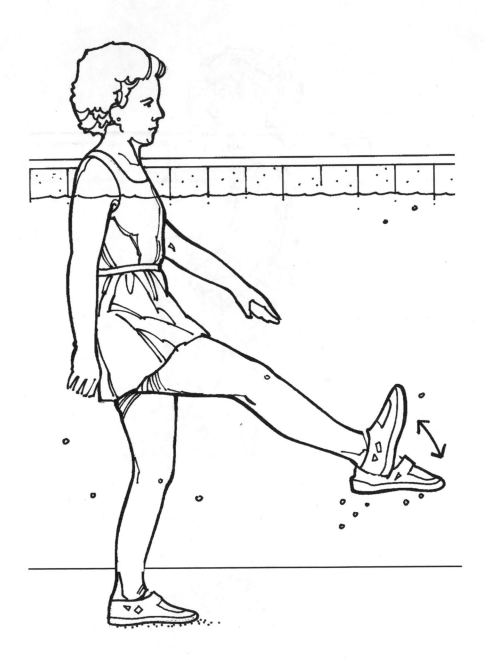

2. ANKLE FLEX

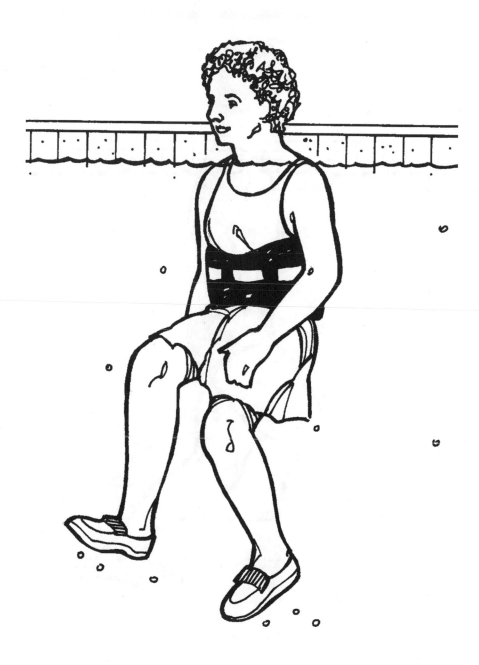

3. BICYCLE

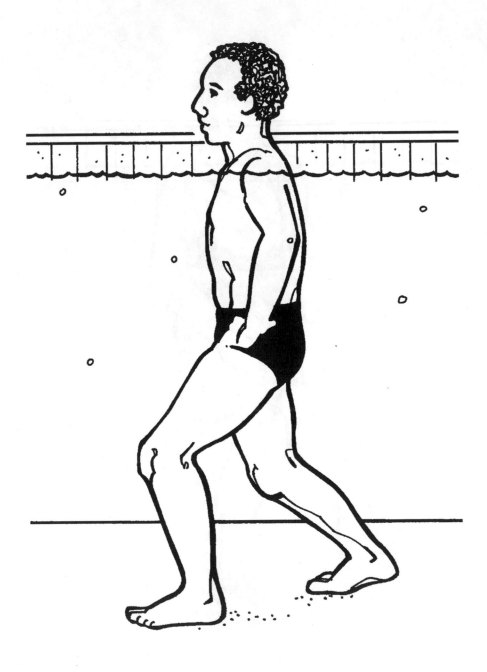

4.   BENT-KNEE WALKING

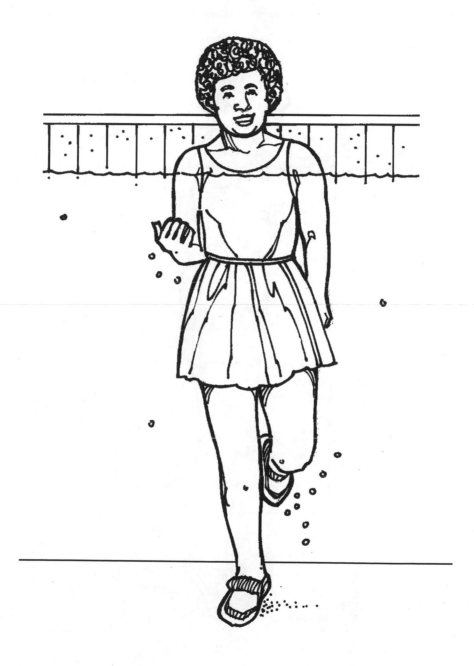

5. BUTTOCK KICK JOG

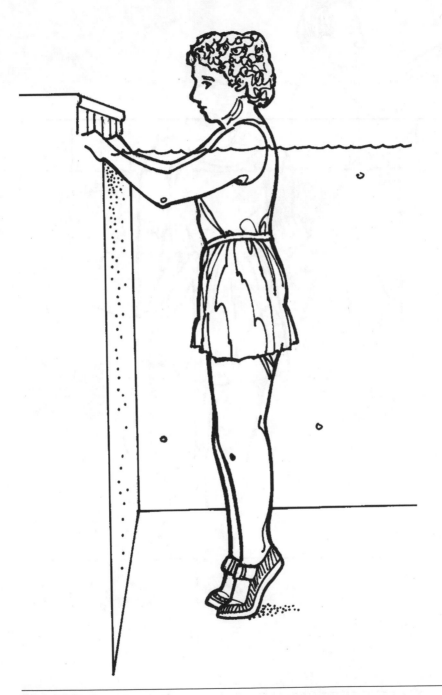

6. CALF

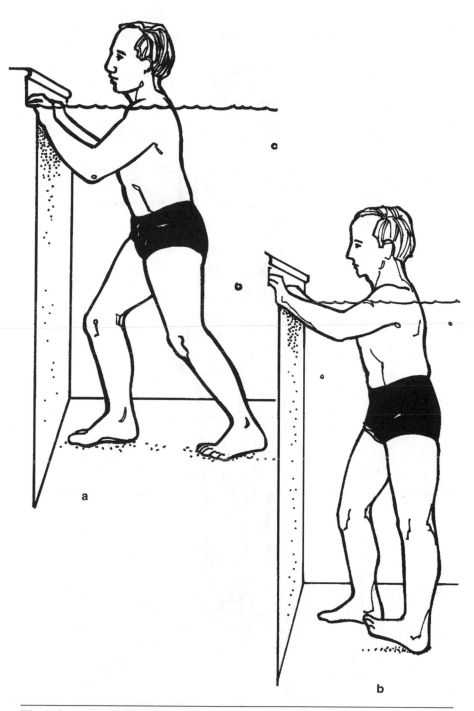

7. CALF STRETCH

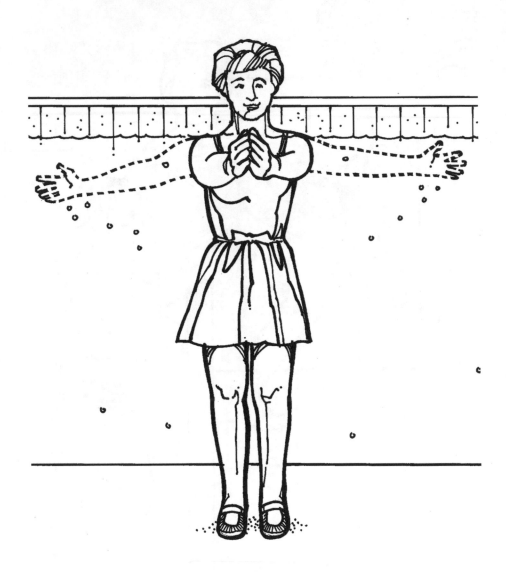

8. CHEST AND UPPER BACK

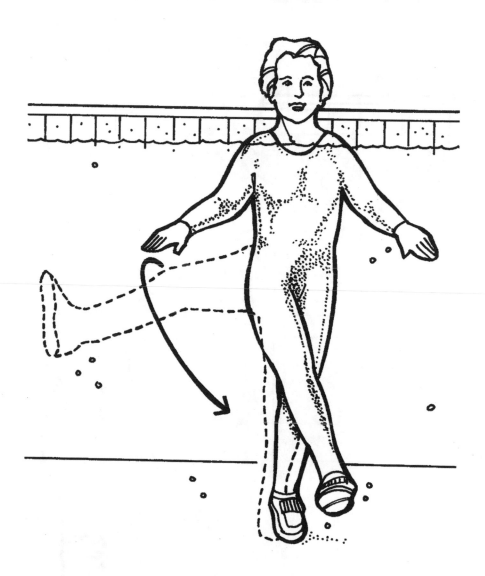

9.   CIRCLE AND STEP

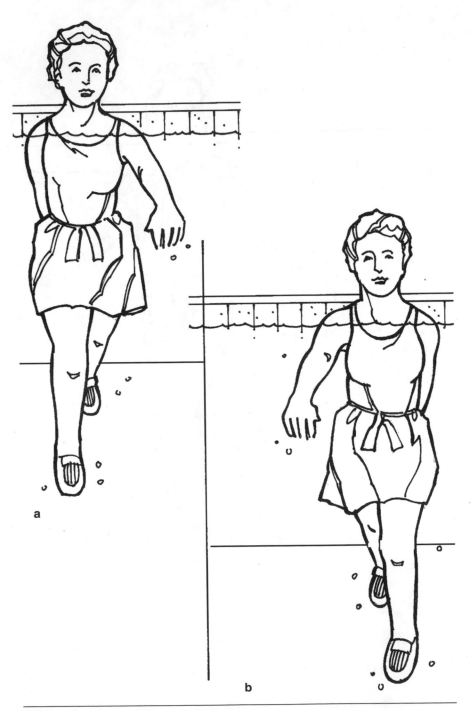

a

b

10. CROSS-COUNTRY SKI

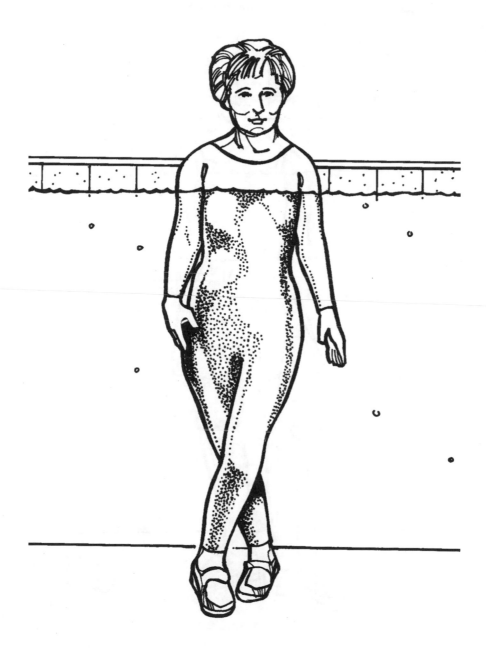

11. CROSSING STEP

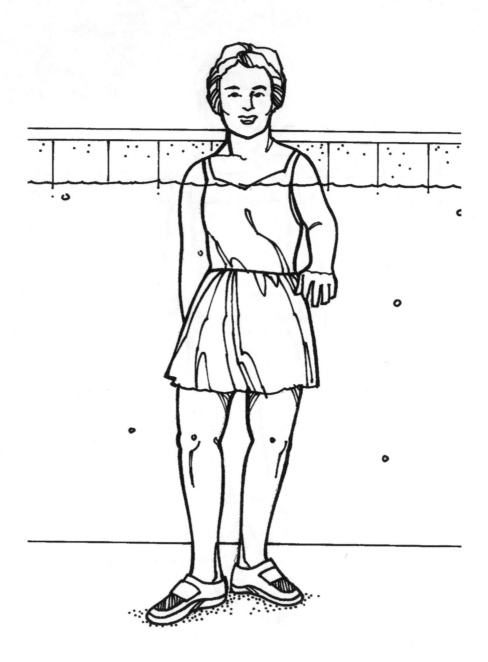

12. DUCK WALK

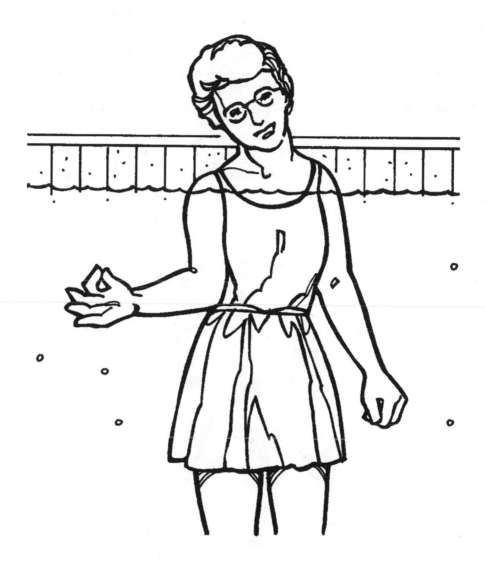

13. FINGER TOUCHES

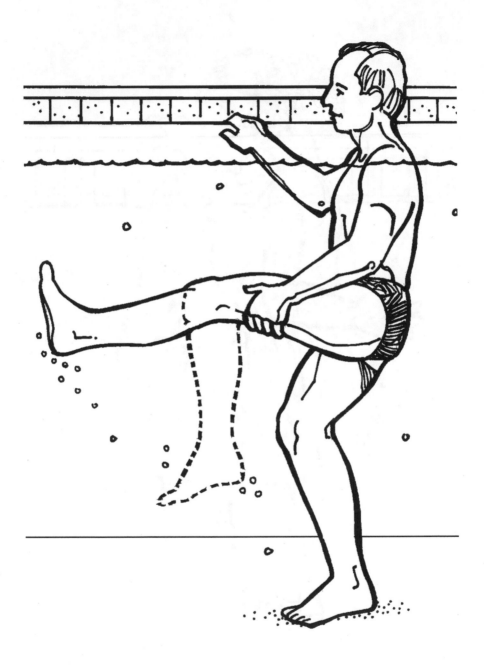

14. FRONT AND BACK OF THIGH

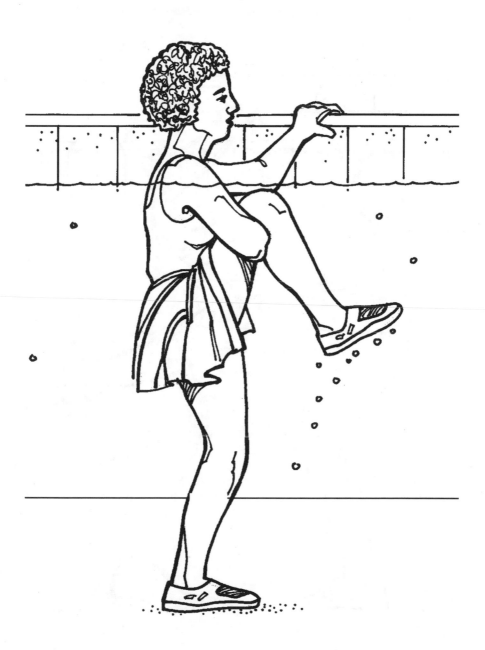

15.   GLUTEAL STRETCH

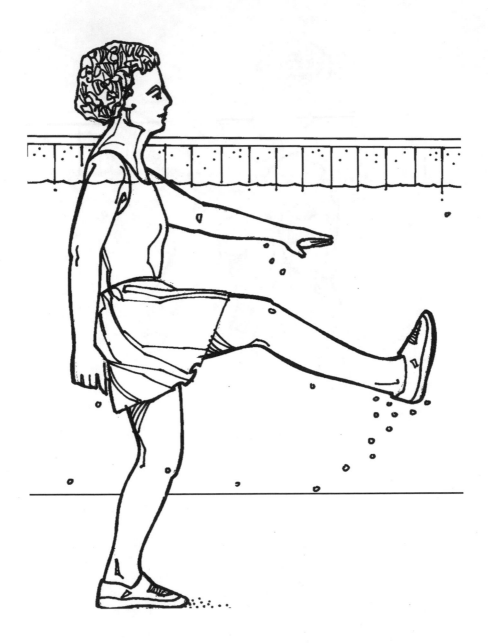

16. GOOSE STEP

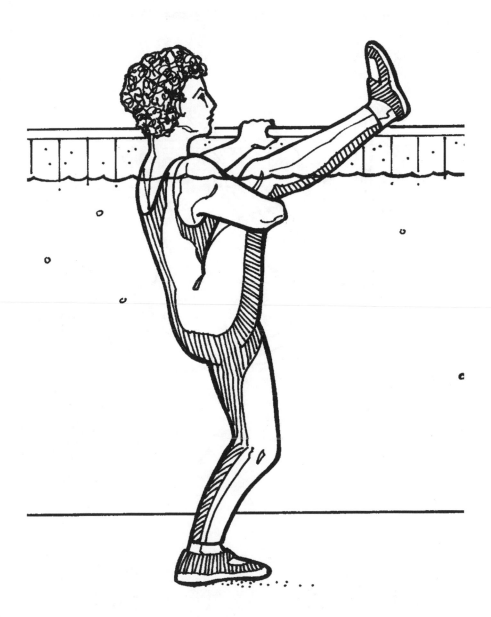

17. HAMSTRING STRETCH—STANDING

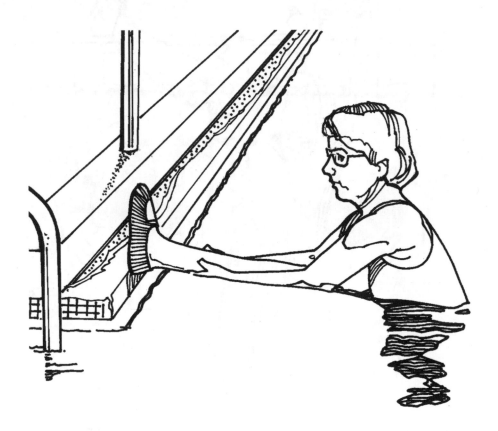

18.   HAMSTRING STRETCH—SUPPORTED LEG

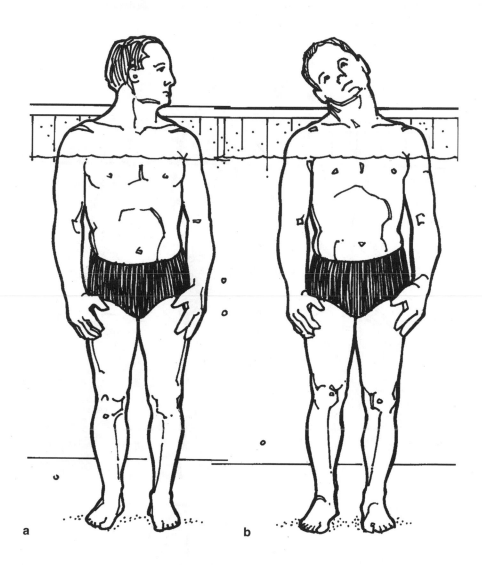

a   b

19. HEAD AND NECK STRETCH—ROLL TO SIDE

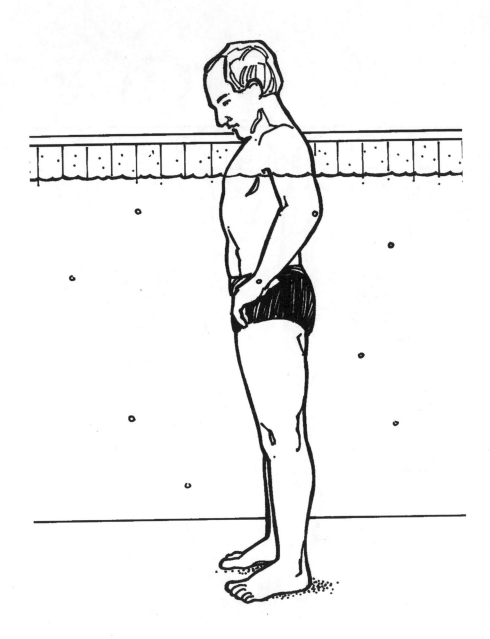

20. HEAD AND NECK STRETCH—ROLL FORWARD

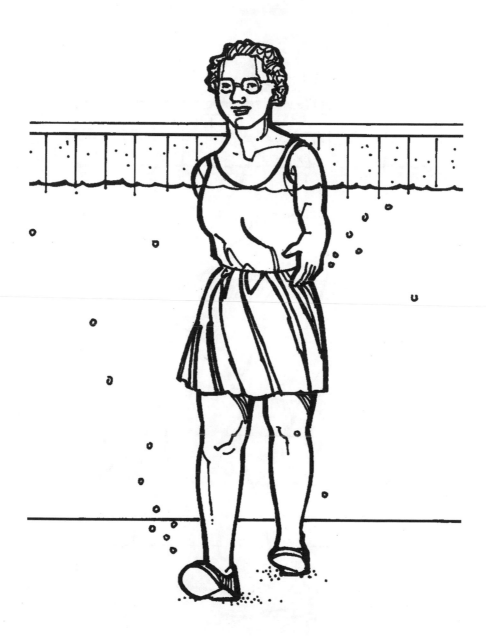

21. HEEL WALKING

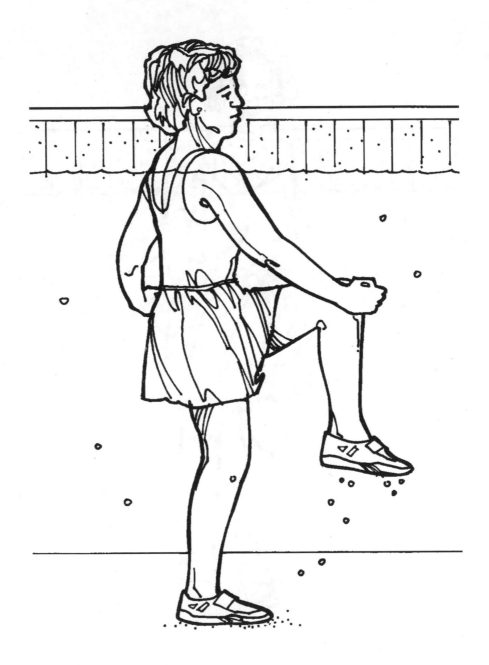

22. HIGH KNEE JOG

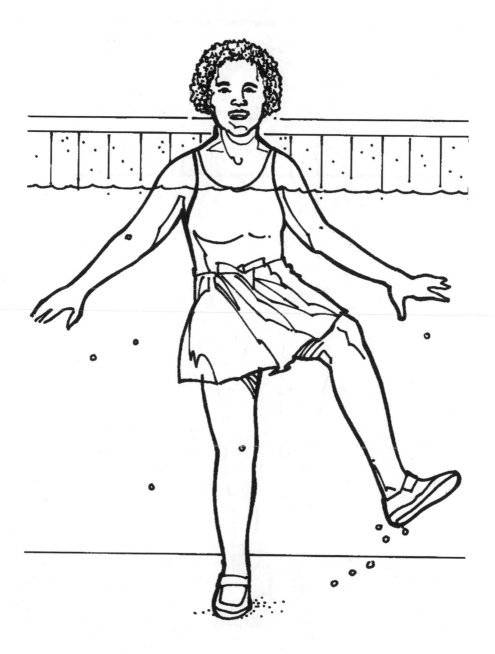

23. HIGH KNEE OUT

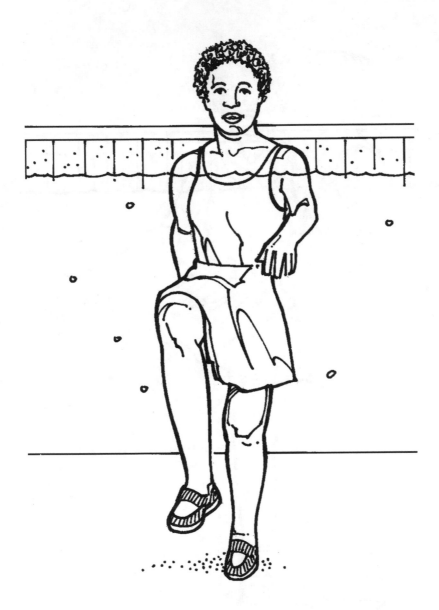

24.   HIGH KNEE STEP

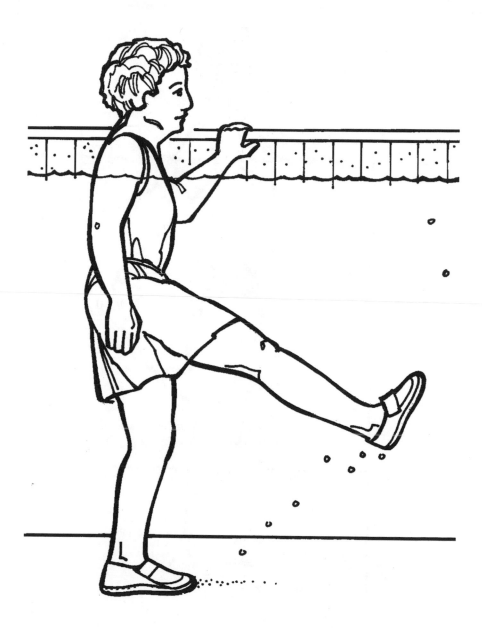

25. HIP AND BUTTOCK

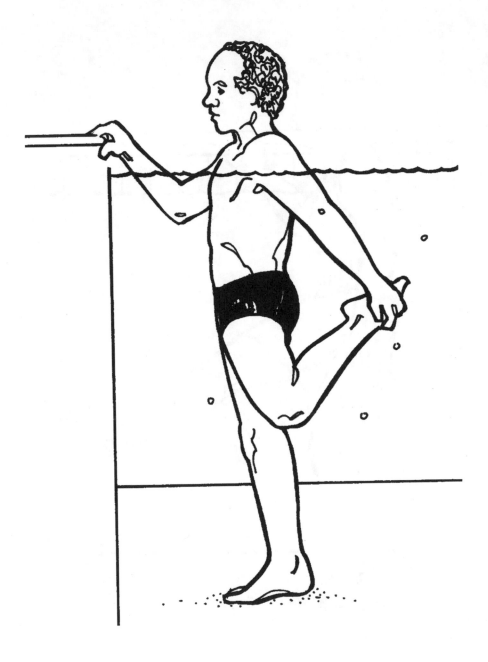

26. HIP FLEXOR STRETCH

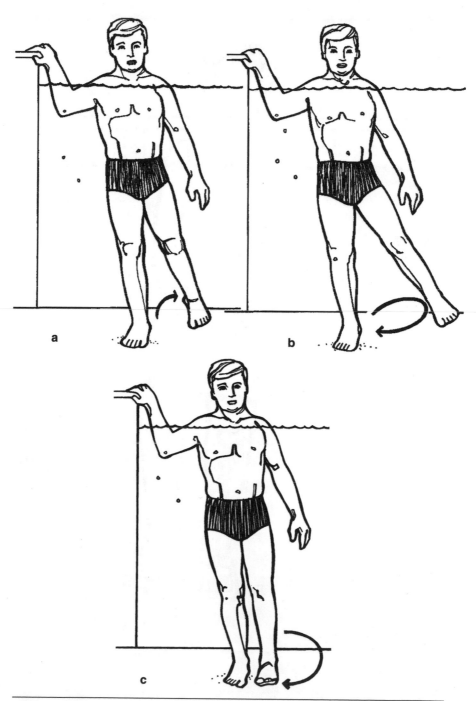

a

b

c

27. HIPS

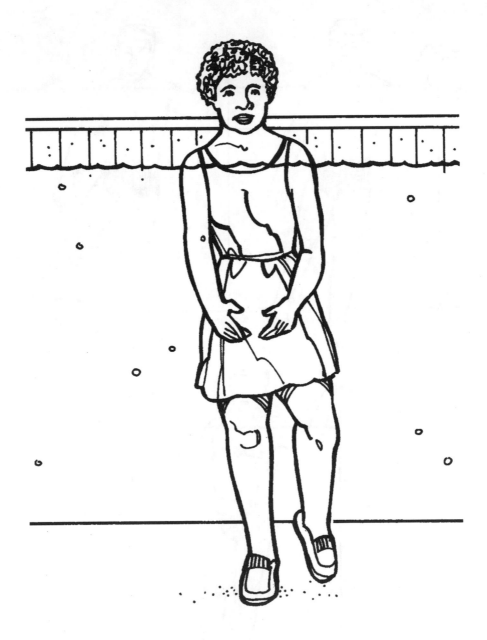

28. HOP

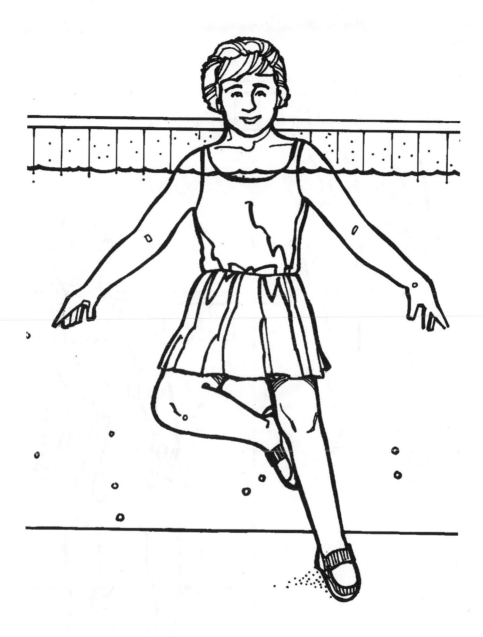

29. HOPSCOTCH

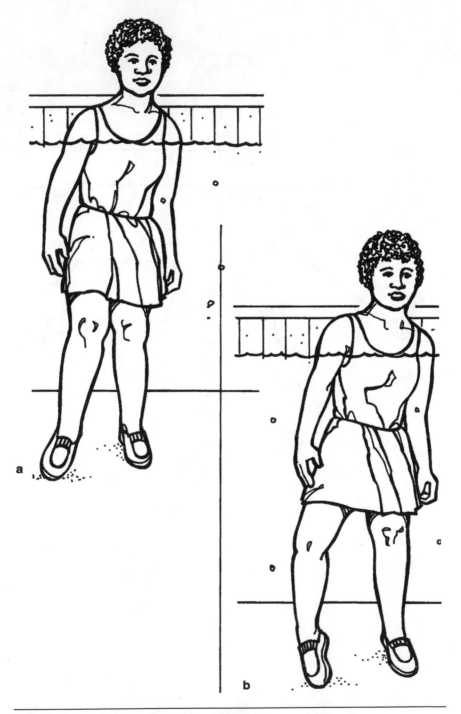

30.   JOINT EXERCISE—ANKLE

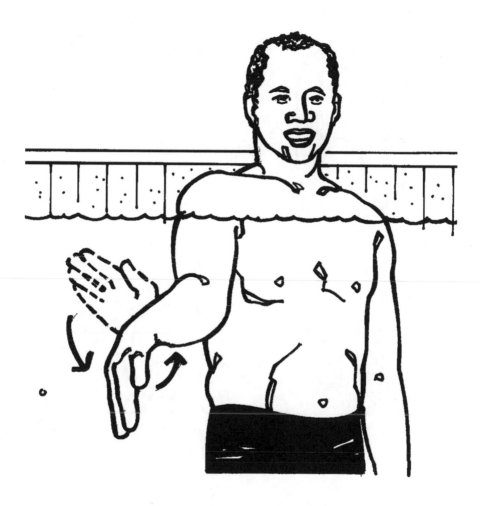

31. JOINT EXERCISE—WRIST

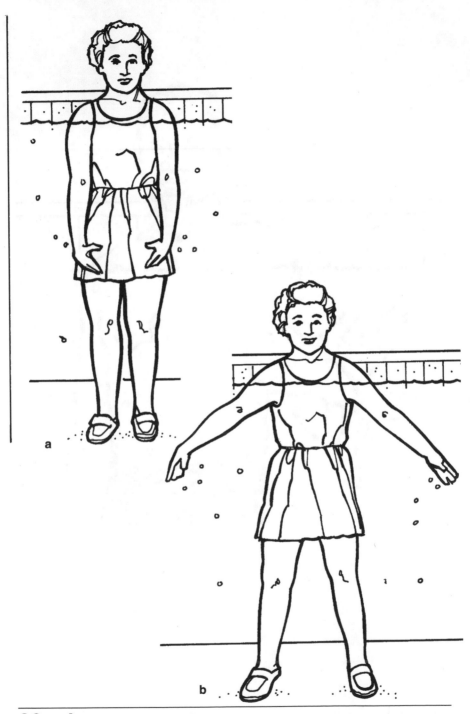

a

b

32.   JUMPING JACKS

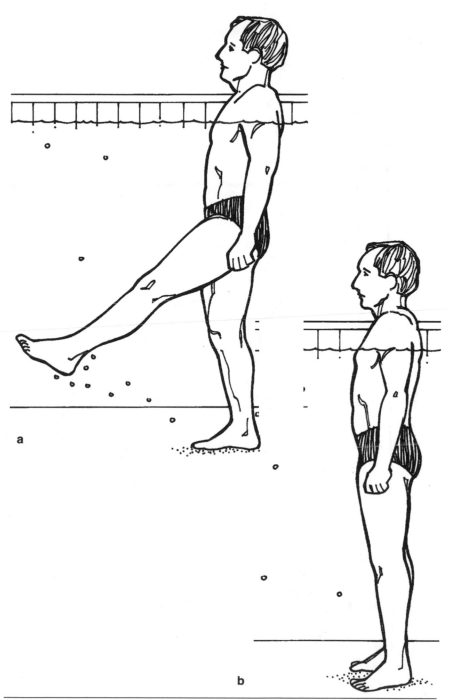

a

b

c

33.   KICK

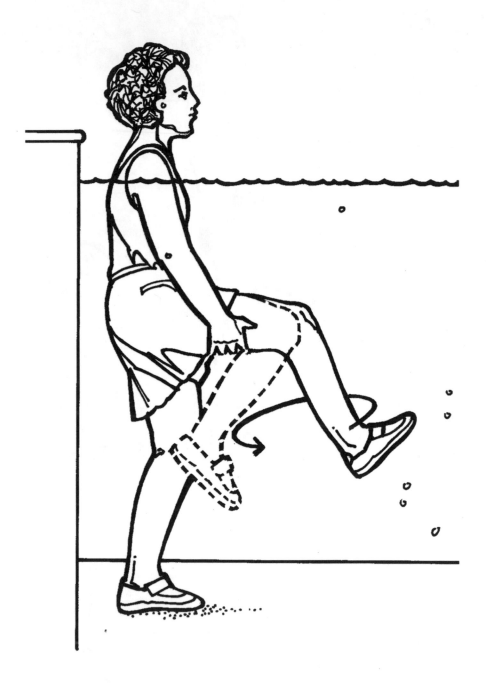

34. KNEE CIRCLES

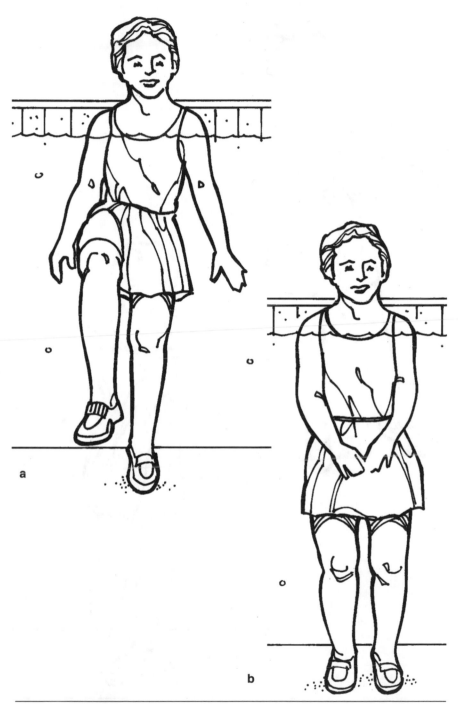

a

b

35. KNEELIFT

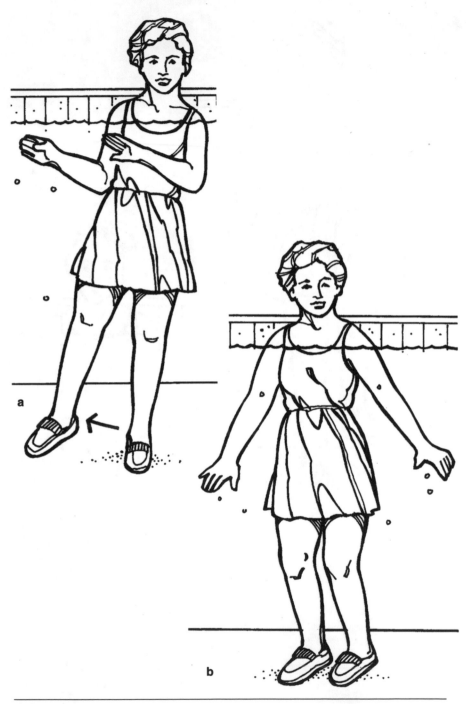

a

b

36. LEAP

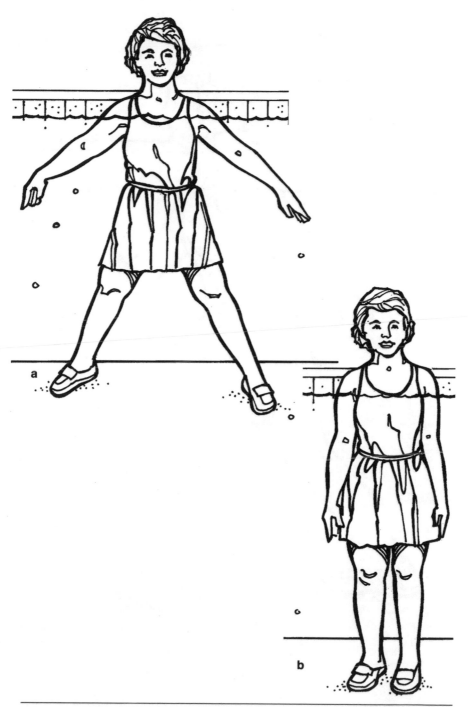

37. LONG-STRIDE SIDE STEP

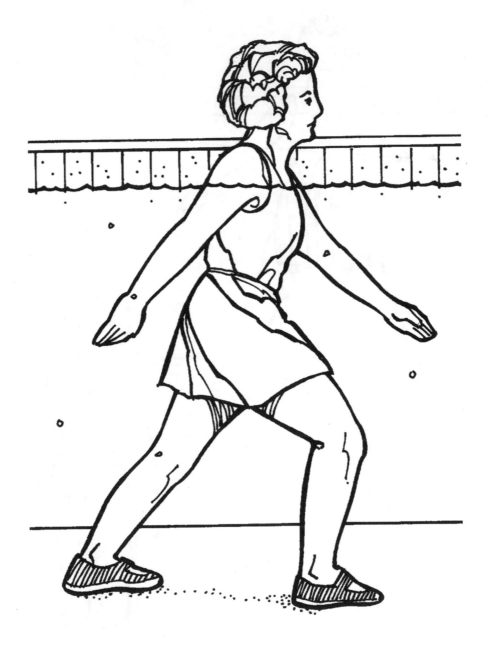

38. LONG-STRIDE WALKING

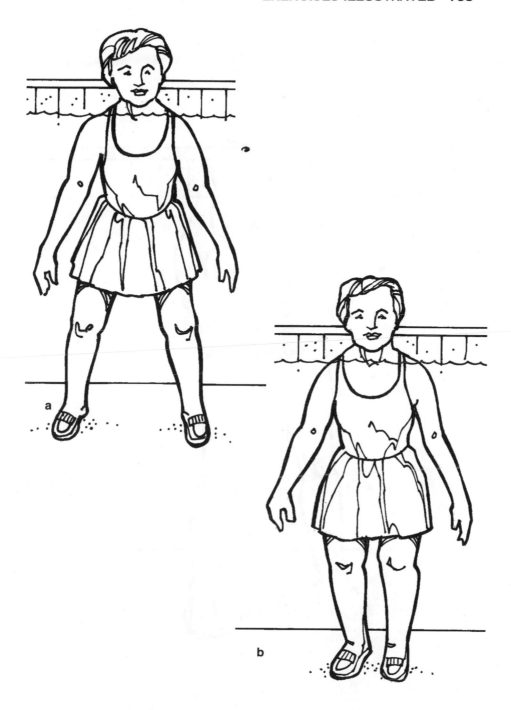

39.   LOW SIDE STEP

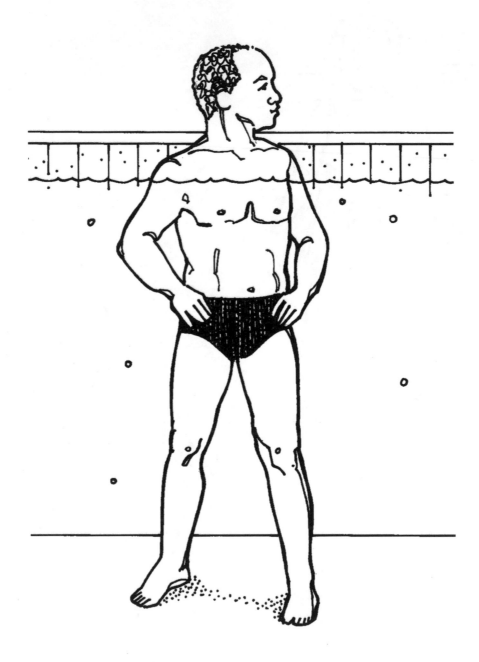

40. MIDRIFF STRETCH

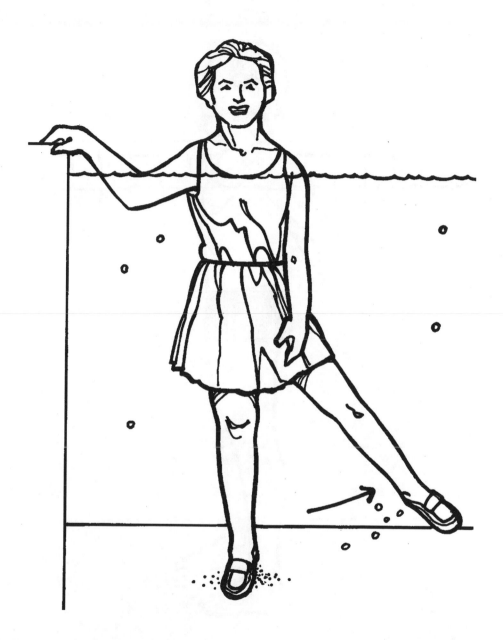

41. OUTER AND INNER THIGH

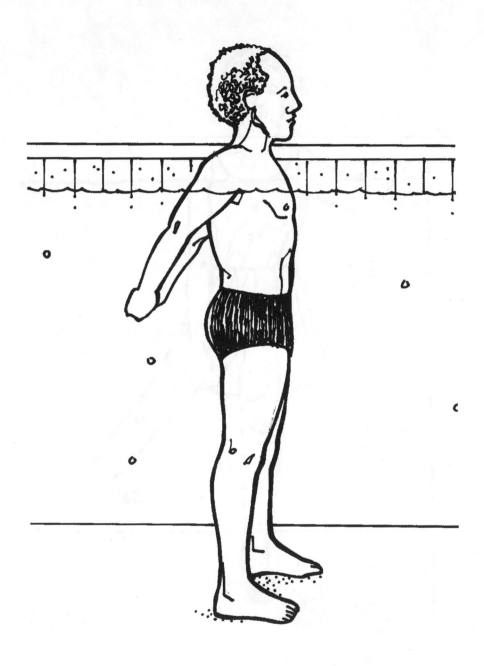

42.   PECTORAL STRETCH—ARMS BACK

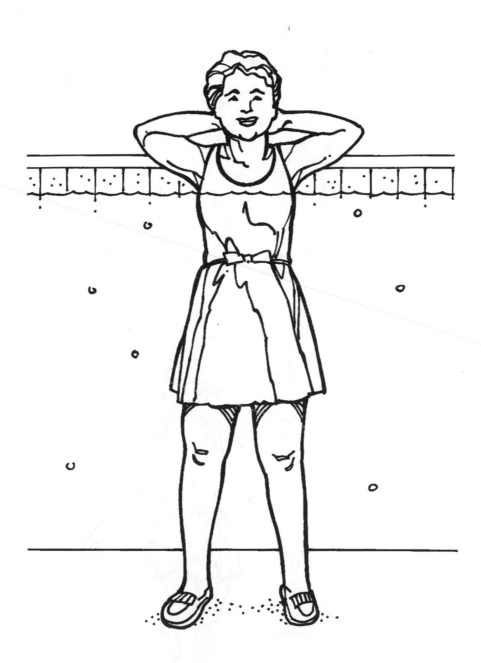

43. PECTORAL STRETCH—ELBOWS OUT

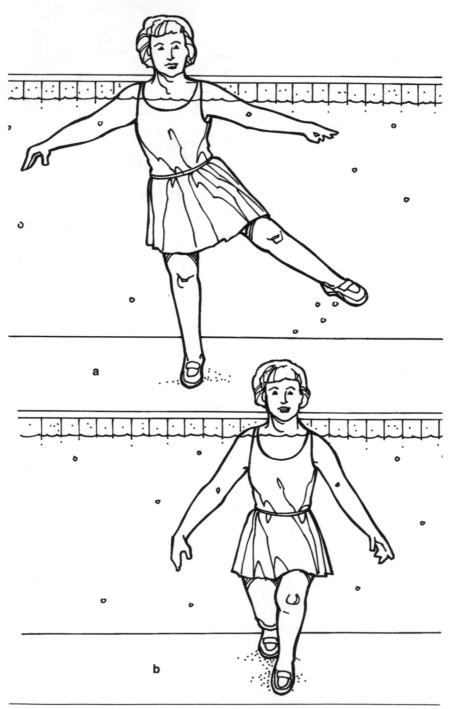

a

b

44.   POWER STEP

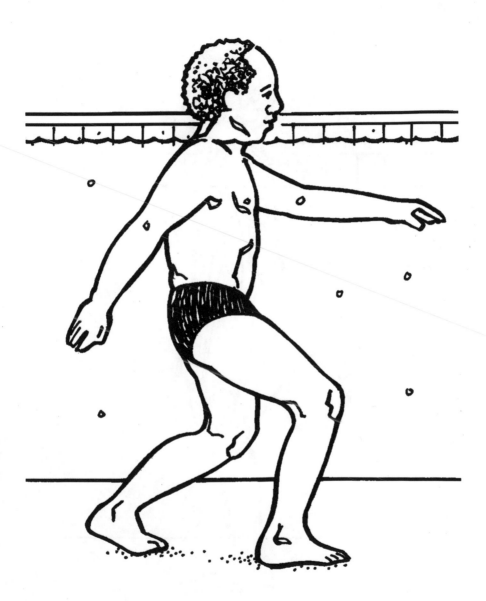

45. POWER WALK

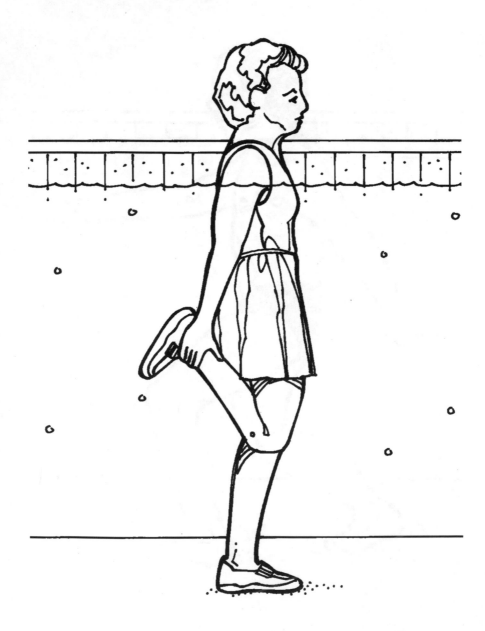

46.   QUADRICEP STRETCH

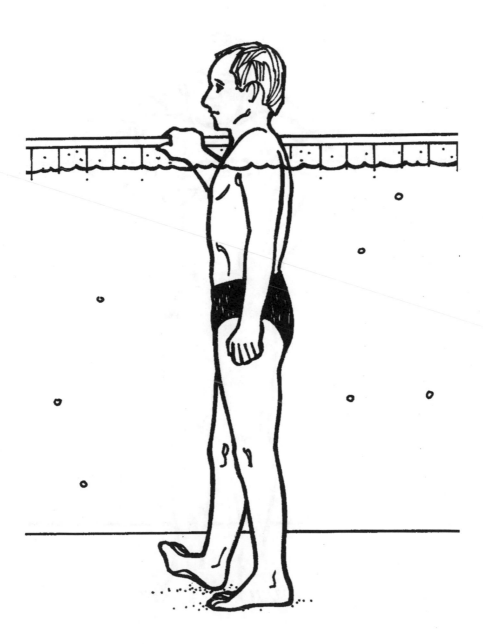

47. SHINS

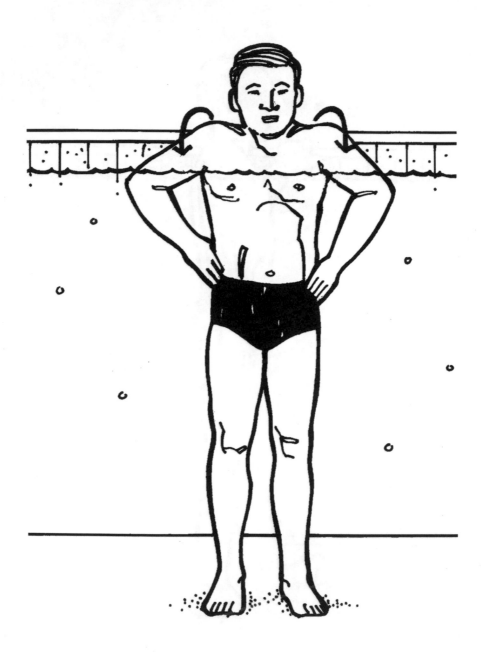

48. SHOULDER ROLLS

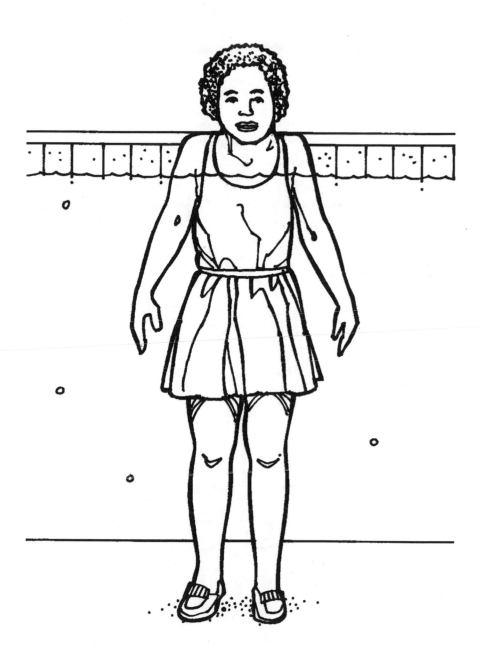

49. SHOULDER SHRUGS

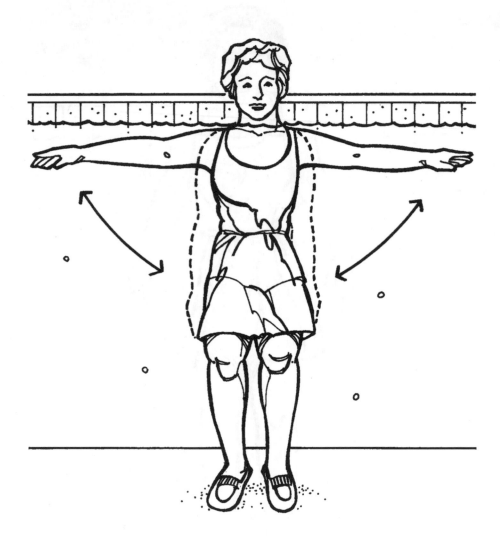

50. SHOULDERS AND SIDES

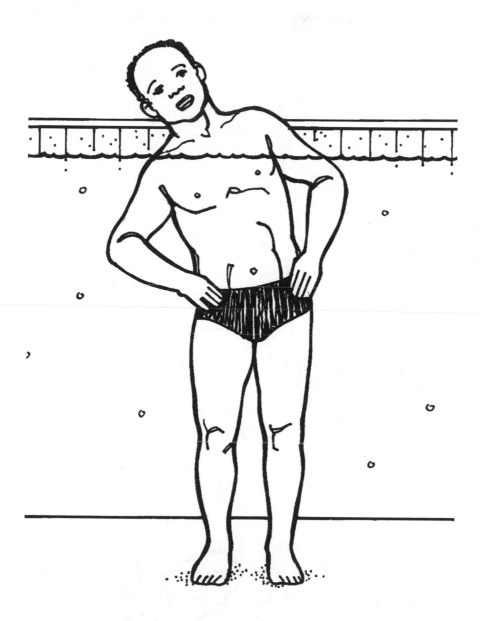

51. SIDE BENDS

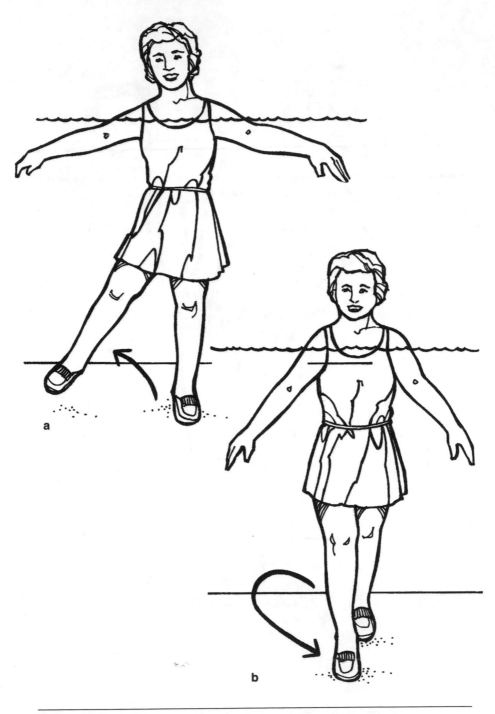

a

b

52. SIDE KICK

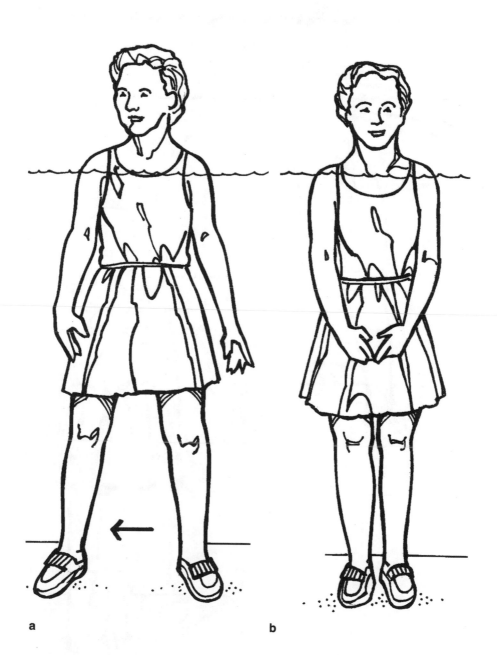

a   b

53. SIDE STEP

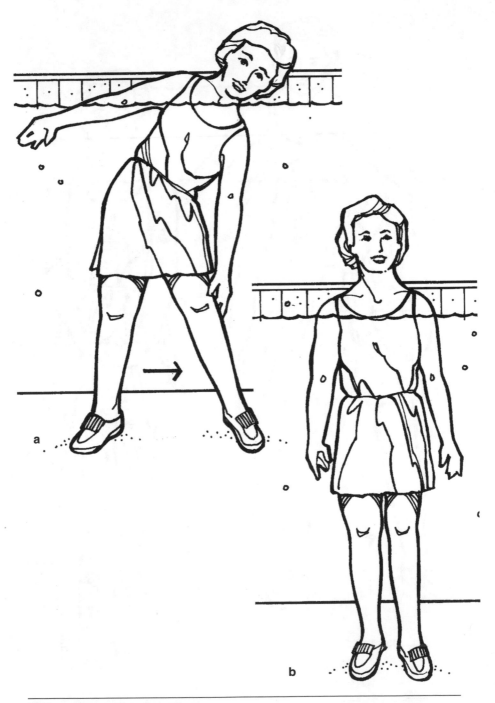

a

b

54. SIDE STEP TILT

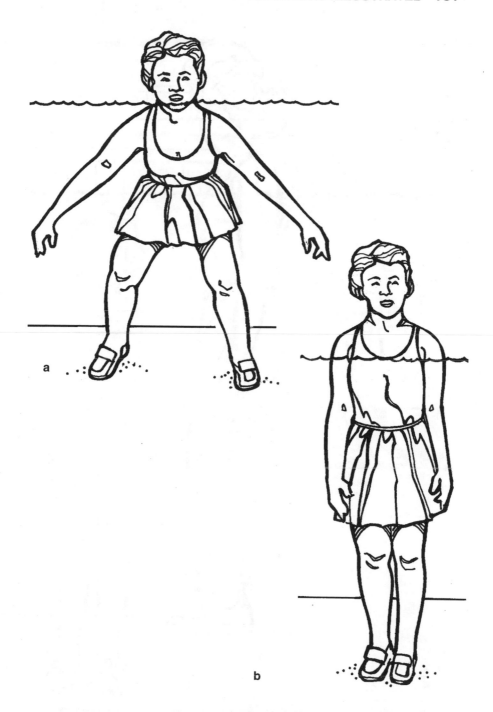

55.   SIDE STEP WITH DIP

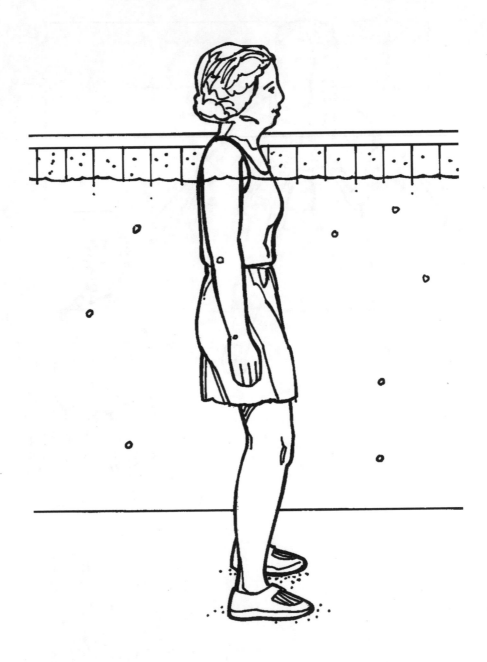

56.   STOMACH

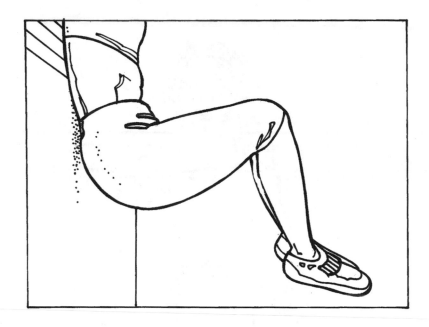

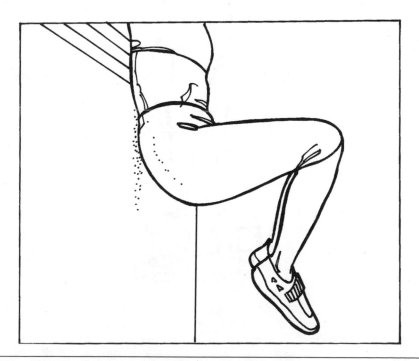

57. STOMACH, MIDRIFF, AND BACK

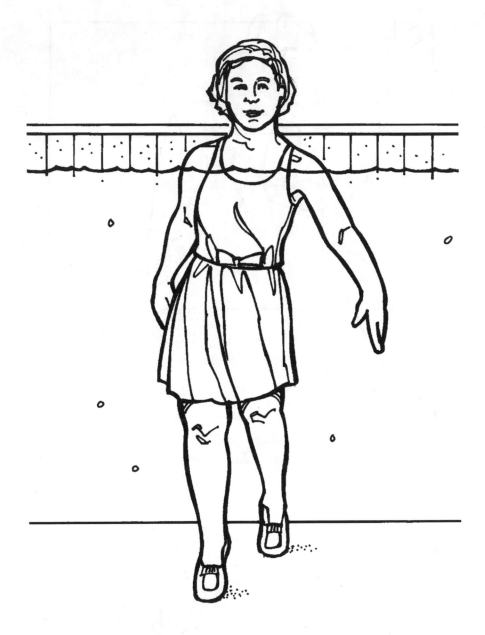

58. TIPTOE WALKING

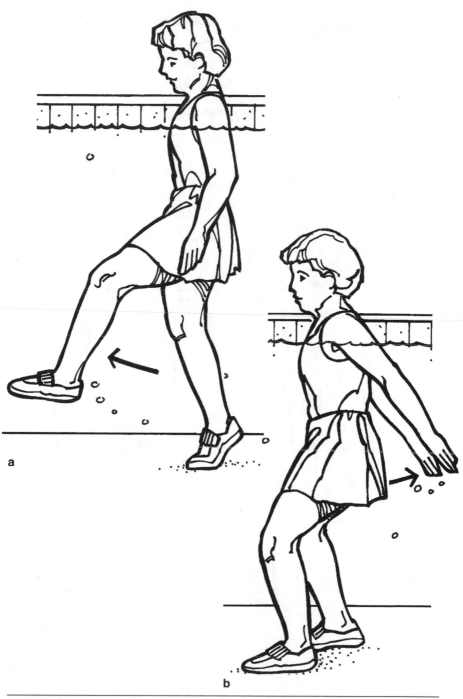

59. TURN AND LEAP

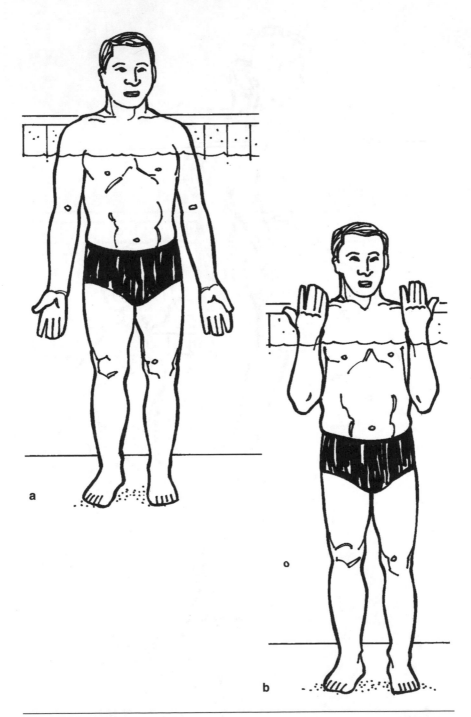

60.   UPPER ARMS

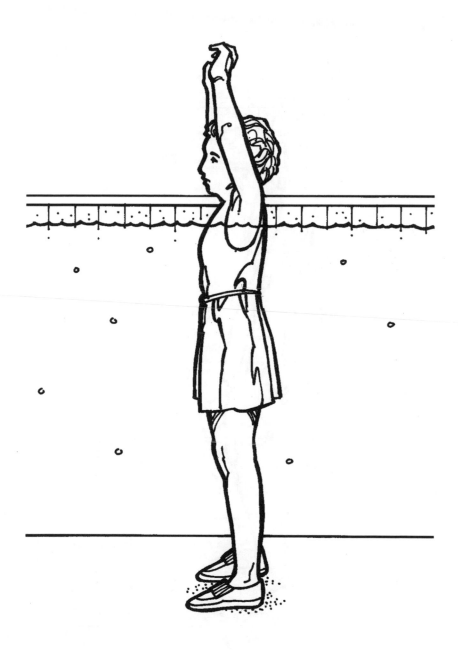

61. UPPER BODY STRETCH—ARMS ABOVE HEAD

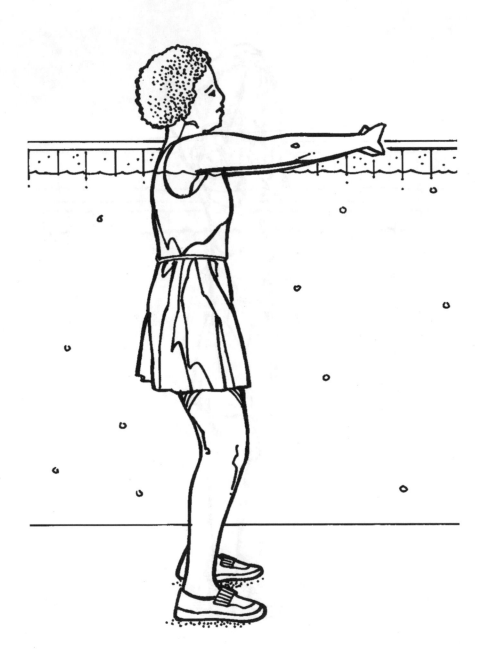

62. UPPER BODY STRETCH—ARMS FORWARD

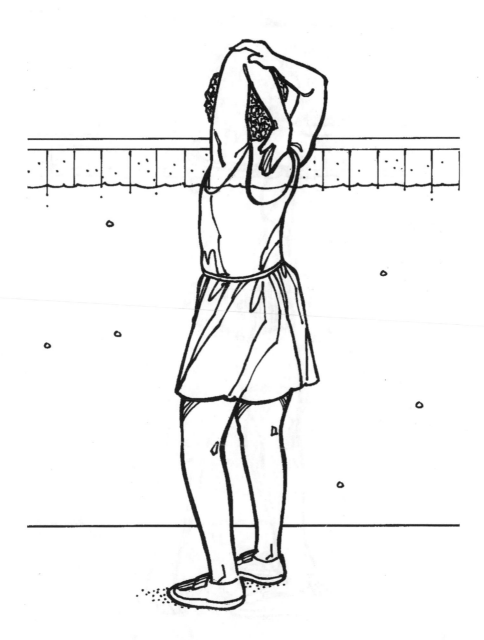

63. UPPER BODY STRETCH—ARM WRAPPED BEHIND

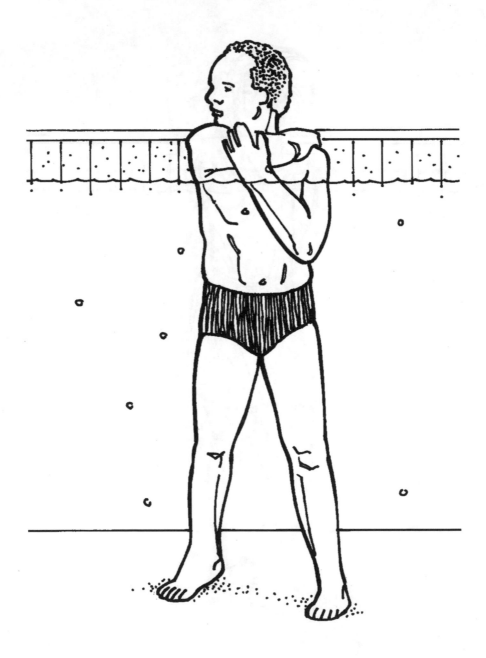

64. UPPER BODY STRETCH—RIGHT ARM WRAPPED

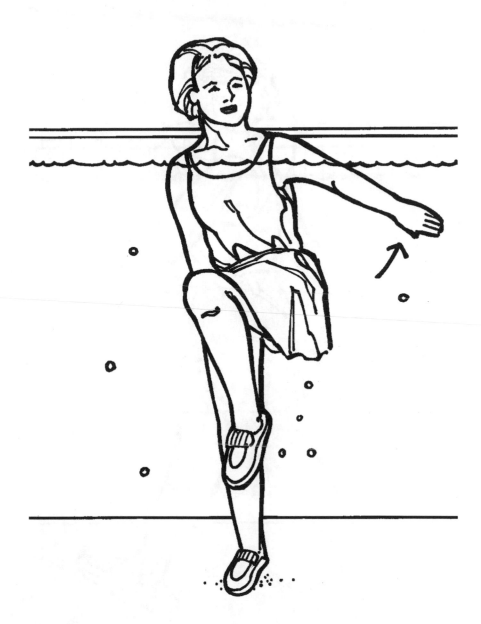

65.   VIGOROUS MOVING HOP

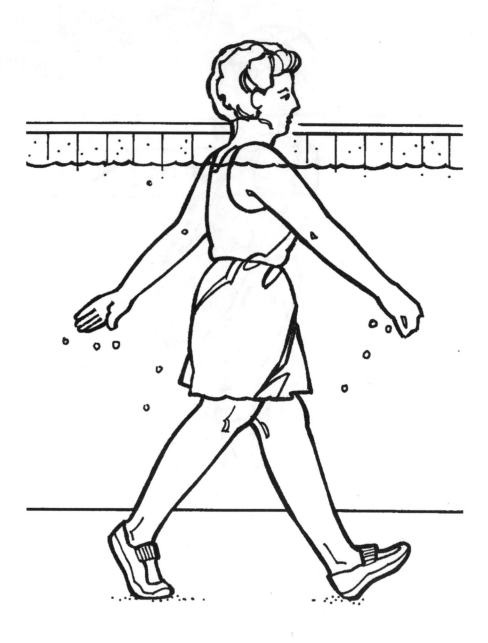

66. WALK AND ROLL—BIG STEP

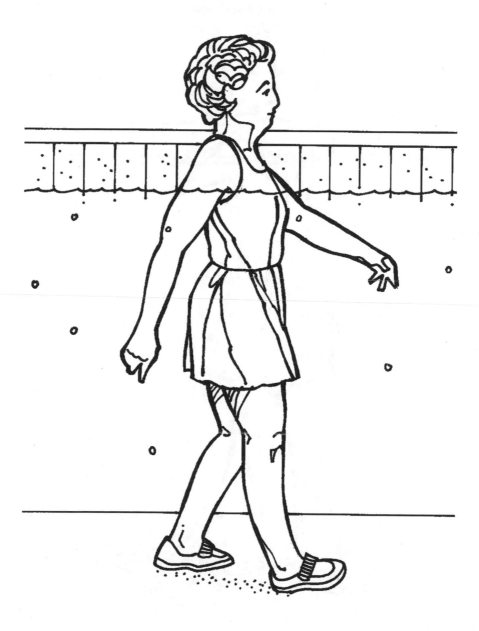

67. WALK AND ROLL—SMALL STEP

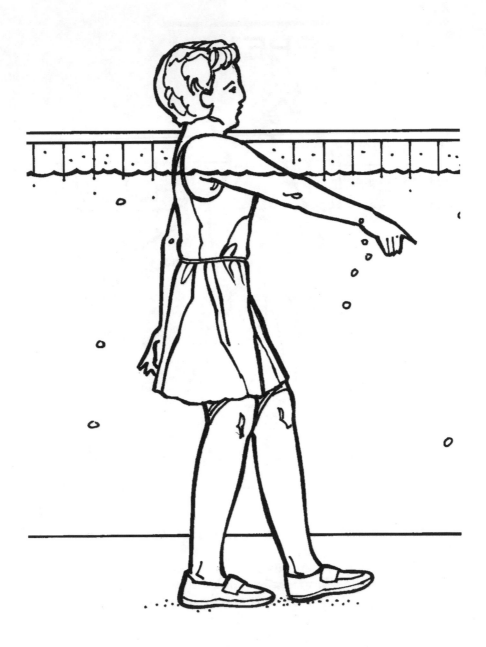

68.   WALKING THE LINE

APPENDIX

RESOURCES

Aquatics Magazine
404-955-2500

6151 Powers Ferry Rd. NW
Atlanta, GA 30339

**Alliance for Food
and Fiber**
310-446-1827

10866 Wilshire Blvd., Suite 550
Los Angeles, CA 90024-4303

A voluntary, nonpolitical association of California farm organizations, individuals, and companies representing about 100,000 farmers and ranchers. It provides information to the public on issues and practices related to the safety and wholesomeness of the food supply.

American Cancer Society
800-ACS-2345

ACS provides consumer information on the link between diet and cancer and on healthy eating plans. Fruits and vegetables provide fiber, vitamins A and C, and more—nutrients thought to lower your risk of developing cancer. Contact your state or local chapter for posters, videos, and other materials.

American Heart Association
214-373-6300

7272 Greenville Ave.
Dallas, TX 75231-4596

AHA produces and distributes print and audiovisual materials for health professionals and the general public, answers inquiries, maintains a resource library and makes referrals to other sources of information.

**American Institute for
Cancer Research Newsletter**

1759 R Street NW
Washington, DC 20077-3618

American Public Health Association
202-789-5600

1015 15th Street NW
Suite 300
Washington, DC 20005

Aquatic Exercise Association
813-486-8600

902 Albee Rd.
P.O. Box 1609
Nokomis, FL 34275

AEA is an international clearinghouse of information with a bimonthly newsletter and a selection of aquatic books, audio cassettes, and videos. They also offer the universal teacher certification program and other educational conferences and programs. The AEA's newsletter, AKWA Letter, is available by subscription.

AQUATICS—The Complete Reference Guide for Aquatic Fitness Professionals
by Ruth Sova
813-486-8600

Aquatic Exercise
Association
902 Albee Rd.
Nokomis, FL 34275

This book is an encyclopedia of aquatic fitness information for professionals. It is the only book available covering both the complete spectrum of the aquatic fitness industry and peripheral disciplines affecting it. AQUATICS covers all the information needed by the aquatic professional to begin a safe, effective, successful aquatic program.

Aquatic Trends, Inc.
Denise Velinsky, Vice President
1-800-296-5496

649 U.S. Highway One
Suite 14
North Palm Beach, FL 33408

Aquatic Trends carries a water workout station for rehabilitation, toning, strengthening, and conditioning.

Arthritis Foundation, Inc.
New Mexico Chapter

P.O. Box 8022
Albuquerque, NM 87198

This group has designed a therapeutic aquatic exercise program for people in constant pain from severe arthritis.

Biosig Instruments, Inc.

5471 Royalmount Ave.
Montreal, PQ H4P1J3

176 Rugar St.
Plattsburg, NY 12901

P.O. Box 860
Champlain, NY 12919

Biosig carries heart rate monitors and biofeedback devices.

Center for the Study of Aging   706 Madison Ave.
518-465-6927   Albany, NY 12208

The center has an extensive list of books available for purchase. Write for a copy of the list, order forms, and more information on the center's activities.

Consumer Information Center   Dept. 314-A
719-948-3334   Pueblo, CO 81009

The 1990 Dietary Guidelines recommend a varied and balanced diet. Suggested daily fruit consumption is 2-4 servings, and suggested vegetable consumption is 3-5 servings a day. Obtain 1-10 free copies by writing to the above address. Ask for Nutrition and Your Health: Dietary Guidelines for Americans, Third Edition, 1990, Home and Garden Bulletin No. 232.

Country Technology, Inc.   P.O. Box 87
608-735-4718   Gays Mills, WI 54631

Vital Signs, a catalog of products for rehabilitation, sports medicine, and physical fitness, is available from Country Technology.

Danmar Products, Inc.   221 Jackson Industrial Dr.
800-783-1998   Ann Arbor, MI 48103

Danmar carries easy-access swimsuits and aquatic exercise aides.

D.K. Douglas Company, Inc.   299 Bliss Rd.
800-334-9070   Longmeadow, MA 01106

D.K. Douglas sells a unique wetsuit vest for warmth during exercise.

Excell Sports Science   450 W. 5th Ave.
503-484-2454   Eugene, OR 97401
Excell Sports sells a water exercise buoyancy belt called the AquaJogger.

50-Plus Athletes Hall of Fame   723 Oakview Dr.
813-756-8808   Bradenton, FL 34210
Accepts nominations for athletes who have made outstanding achievements in their favorite sport after their 50th birthday.

Fitness Wholesale   895-A Hampshire Rd.
800-537-5512   Stow, OH 44224

Fitness Wholesale carries numerous products for use in aquatic exercise.

Food & Nutrition   National Agricultural Library
Information Center   Room 304
                                                    10301 Baltimore Blvd.
                                                    Beltsville, MD 20705

Provides audiovisual and print materials for consumers and professionals on topics in human nutrition, foodservice management, and food technology. Part of USDA.

Food Watch   Agriculture Council of America
202-682-9200   927 15th NW, Ste. 800
                                                    Washington, DC 20005

A full-scale, nationwide public education and awareness program to build public confidence in the food and fiber industry. Has an Information Center that can answer your food safety questions.

HydroFit   405 Lincoln St.
800-346-7295   Eugene, OR 97401

Makers of aquatic fitness gear. Call for free catalogue.

Aquatic Connections/Hydro-Tone   P.O. Box 556
International, Inc.   Lakeland, MI 48143
810-231-0836

Hydro-Tone sells equipment that increases water resistance during a water workout.

Hydrophonics   880 Calle Plano, Unit J
805-383-7522   Camarillo, CA 93012

Hydrophonics sells the Swimman Waterproof Personal Stereo Systems that allow you to listen to music or exercise tapes while exercising in the water.

INFOFIT   Katherine MacKeigan
Leisure Management and Education   10814 75th Ave.
                                                    Edmonton, AB T6E1K2

J & B Foam Fabricators, Inc.   P.O. Box 144
800-621-3626   Ludington, MI 49431

J & B Foam Fabricators sells foam belts, discs, and barbells for use in water exercise classes. Call for free catalog.

National Health Information Clearinghouse   P.O. Box 1133
800-336-4797   Washington, DC 20013-1133

Answers consumer and health professional's inquiries, operates telephone "hotline" service, produces and distributes print materials for professionals as well as the general public. Develops computerized databases, maintains a resource library, makes referrals to other sources of information, and provides reference services.

National Heart, Lung, and Blood   P.O. Box 30105
Information Center   Bethesda, MD 20824-0105
301-251-1222

Information support activity of the National Cholesterol Education Program and the National High Blood Pressure Education Program. Consumer education materials on cholesterol and sodium are available. Scientific materials are available for professionals.

Outreach Diabetes Education for Georgia   1467 Harper St.
Division of Endocrine Disease   HB 5025
706-733-0188 Ext. 2171 (Voice Mail)   Medical College of Georgia
706-721-2131   Augusta, GA 30912

Anne Whittington-Reardon, RN, MSN, CDE, is a certified diabetes educator. She is available to answer questions about diabetes.

Sprint/Rothhammer International, Inc.   P.O. Box 5579
800-235-2156   Santa Maria, CA 93456

Sprint/Rothhammer offers numerous water-related products.

Strom-Berg Productions   253 Rhodes Ct.
408-295-3898   San Jose, CA 95126

Strom-Berg sells music for use in aquatic exercise programs.

United States Senior Athletic Games   200 Castlewood Dr.
Manya Joyce, President   North Palm Beach, FL 33408

U.S. National Senior   14323 S. Outer Forty Rd., Ste. N300
Sports Organization   Chesterfield, MO 63017
314-878-4900

Promotes fitness and physical excellence through competition among adults 55 and over. Establishes local and regional senior games throughout the U.S. and organizes the U.S. National Senior Olympics.

Washington, DC:

Administration on Aging
Alliance for Aging Research
American Association of Retired Persons
Congressional Committees
    House Select Committee on Aging
    Senate Aging Committee
    Senate Majority Special Committee on Aging
    Senate Minority Special Committee on Aging
Pepper Commission

YMCA Program Store   Box 5077
217-351-5076   Champaign, IL 61820
800-747-0089

YMCA carries the More New Games Book. The New Games philosophy is "Everybody Wins, Nobody Loses." These games are ideal for water exercise.

Young Enterprises, Inc.   107 N. Main
913-727-2263   Lansing, KS 66043

Developed a land-based program of wellness for older adults.

BIBLIOGRAPHY

American College of Sports Medicine. (1982). *Guidelines for graded exercise testing and exercise prescription.* Indianapolis: Author.

American Council on Exercise. (1991). *Personal trainer manual,* M. Sudy (Ed.). San Diego: Author.

American Heart Association. (1989). *1989 heart facts.* Dallas: Author.

Antihypertensives and exercise conditioning. (1990). *The Physician and Sportsmedicine,* **18**(9), 24.

Bedgood, D.H. (1988). Bones in the pool. *The AKWA Letter,* **1**(6), 1-3.

Chossek, V., Delzeit, L., Lindle, J., Sova, R., & Windhorst, M. (1990). *Aquatic concepts.* Port Washington, WI: Aquatic Exercise Association.

Goldstein, E.E., Simkin, A., Epstein, L., Peritz, E. (1994, winter). The influence of weight-bearing water exercises on bone density of postmenopausal women. *H₂Oz News,* 10-11.

IDEA Foundation. (1987). *Aerobic Dance-Exercise Instructor Manual.* San Diego, CA: Author.

Ike, M., Lampman, W., & Castor, S. (1989). Arthritis and aerobic exercise: A review. *The Physician and Sportsmedicine,* **17**(2), 47.

Reebok. (1990). *Reebok instructor news* (vol. 3, no. 4). Dallas: Institute for Aerobics Research.

Rikli, R., & McManis, B. (1990). Effects of exercise on bone mineral content in postmenopausal women. *Research Quarterly for Exercise and Sport,* **61**(3), 243-249.

Van Camp, G., & Boyer, B. (1989). Exercise guidelines for the elderly. *The Physician and Sportsmedicine,* **17**(5), 14-16.

Welch, D. (1989, July). Water dancing. *Health,* 46-51.

Young, T. *Older adult exercise manual.* Lansing, KS: Young Enterprises.

INDEX

Note: Page numbers in italics refer to tables and figures.

ABOUT THE AUTHOR

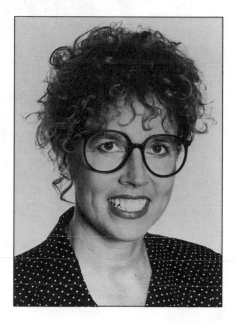

Ruth Sova, MS, is an internationally recognized leader in the health and fitness industry. Considered the world's foremost expert on aquatic fitness, she is founder and past-president of the Aquatic Exercise Association and president of the Aquatic Therapy and Rehabilitation Institute.

Sova is author of 70 articles and several books on aquatic exercise for fitness instructors, including *Aquatics: The Complete Guide for Aquatic Fitness Professionals*, *Aquatic Exercise*, and *The Aquatic Activities Handbook*. She is winner of the first Presidential Sports Award in aquatic exercise, and recipient of the IDEA Outstanding Business Award, and the Aquatic Exercise Association's Contribution to the Aquatics Industry Award. Sova is also a member of the American Alliance for Health, Physical Education, Recreation and Dance; the Council for National Cooperation in Aquatics; and the Wisconsin Governor's Council on Physical Fitness.

Sova has conducted hundreds of clinics across the country and continues to write, teach, and speak on wellness and aquatic activities. She lives with her husband, Bud, in Port Washington, Wisconsin.

Full Life Fitness

A Complete Exercise Program for Mature Adults

Janie Clark, MA

1992 • Paper • 192 pp
Item PCLA0391 • ISBN 0-87322-391-8
$13.95 ($17.50 Canadian)

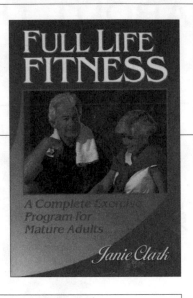

Full Life Fitness will help older adults enjoy the benefits of physical exercise while avoiding the fatigue and overexertion associated with many exercise plans. It features only low-stress and no-stress exercises designed to help avoid pulled muscles, undue soreness, overtaxed joints, and excess fatigue.

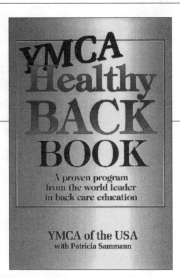

YMCA Healthy Back Book

YMCA of the USA

with Patricia Sammann

1994 • Paper • 120 pp
Item PYMC0629 • ISBN 0-87322-629-1
$10.95 ($15.50 Canadian)

This book contains the most up-to-date, practical information available from the YMCA—an organization that has helped over 300,000 people find relief from back pain. Featuring more than 80 full-color illustrations, a reader-friendly format, and 29 proven back exercises, the *YMCA Healthy Back Book* will help you conquer back problems and return to an active lifestyle.

To place order: U.S. customers call **TOLL-FREE 1 800 747-4457;** customers outside of U.S. use the appropriate telephone number/address shown in the front of this book.

Prices are subject to change.

 Human Kinetics
The Premier Publisher for Sports & Fitness

2335